Mom Mindset Mastery
Igniting Your
Superconscious Swagger

Amanda Maloney

Mom Mindset Mastery: Igniting Your Superconscious Swagger

Mom Mindset Mastery: Igniting Your Superconscious Swagger is published in Garamond with chapter headers in Comic Sans MS.

DEDICATION

To my beautiful mother and sister (the Cuddy girls), thank you for your endless love, support, and wisdom as I navigate motherhood, and to my beloved late father, thank you for instilling in me the confidence to embrace my life's journey. Your years of guidance continue to inspire me every day.

For my husband, my soul mate and partner in crime, your love and support mean the world to me. I could not have done this without you.

To my children, Michael and Sarah, you have opened my heart to a level I never knew existed until I became your mom. Know you are cherished beyond measure and your potential is limitless.

CONTENTS

INTRODUCTION

Welcome to the wild ride of motherhood, where chaos and joy intertwine like a beautiful, messy dance. As a certified Magnetic Mind Coach, wife, and proud mother of two teenagers, I have learned to master the art of not yelling at my kids (well, not as often as I used to), and I can genuinely affirm that I'm living a life I love, filled with purpose and a sprinkle of Superconscious Swagger.

Although it wasn't always this way. Life as a mother felt like a never-ending roller coaster, a chaotic mix of ups and downs. From frantic school drop-offs and rushing to work to juggling sports practices and the perpetual hunt for my phone (which inevitably seemed to disappear into the black hole I called my purse), I was always grappling with the challenges of motherhood that tested my patience and resilience at every turn.

After the birth of my second child, I left the corporate world and embarked on a journey filled with various part-time jobs. Regrettably, financial hardships were our constant companions for years to come. I clung to the hope that every sacrifice made would lay the foundation for my kids' future success and happiness, although, behind the scenes, worry kept me up at night. Were my kids doing well at school? Did they fit in with their friends? Were they making choices that wouldn't make me question my parenting skills?

Cue the social media scroll, where a curated depiction of other moms' perfect lives constantly reminded me of my own shortcomings. The images of seemingly flawless families on amazing vacations and engaging in Pinterest-worthy activities haunted my feeds, making me feel like the underdog in the Motherhood Olympics. The weight of these expectations, our financial woes, and lack of sleep turned me into a frustrated yeller desperately seeking an exit from this overwhelming cycle.

When my kids were 11 and eight, I reentered the workforce full-time to improve our financial situation. Having been out of the office environment for eight years, I settled on a lower-level position with a pay rate to match. My husband worked remotely two days per week at the time. However, for the remaining three days, I found myself juggling work, sports, activities, school events, and appointments with only two weeks of vacation per year. Consequently, the additional income was absorbed by the cost of extracurricular activities to keep our kids occupied during school breaks and summers while I was at work. I was overwhelmed, frustrated, burned out and left with little patience to spare.

Then, things took a turn for the worse. The pandemic struck in 2020, bringing the world to a standstill. Like countless other parents, we found ourselves struggling with the challenge of balancing work responsibilities, assisting our kids with remote schooling, and ensuring the well-being of our family during such uncertain times. Meanwhile, I continued to report to the office.

Determined to maintain stability within our household amidst the uncertainty, I searched for positive mindset techniques online. During this search, I stumbled upon an advertisement for something called a Superconscious Recode, which sparked my curiosity. Intrigued by the possibilities, I enrolled as a client in the Magnetic Mind Masterclass Program, an experience that transformed my life. Motivated by this profound change, I pursued certification in this remarkable practice and can proudly declare that I'm navigating the whirlwind of teenagerhood with a newfound sense of Superconscious Swagger. The black hole in my purse may still exist, but at least I've upgraded from yelling at my kids to a more refined form of communication called eye-rolling.

With the Magnetic Mind Program's invaluable guidance and the insights and strategies I've acquired throughout my own research and experiences, I've discovered the secrets to creating a life I love! I look forward to sharing this transformative journey with other exceptional mothers, spreading joy, and empowering them to embrace their unique paths to fulfillment. So, if you're ready to learn how to shift your mindset and start living a life you love, I'd be honored to be your guide.

There are so many valuable takeaways in this book you can begin implementing today. However, if you'd like to take your journey to the next level, I've also created a course utilizing the Magnetic Mind Method with amazing client feedback. As gratitude for your interest in this book, you can receive **25% off the full-price course** *Learn How to Manifest and Live a Life You Love.* Please visit the Course page on my website below and enter this promo code at checkout: **1BOOK25**

AbundantTransformationsLLC.com

PART 1

Reclaim Your Sanity: Control Your Day with Superconscious Action

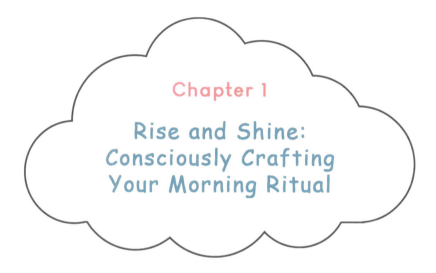

Chapter 1

Rise and Shine: Consciously Crafting Your Morning Ritual

Welcome to the dawn of your transformation! In this chapter, we brew up a morning ritual that sets the tone for a day filled with Superconscious Swagger. Picture this: you, your favorite morning beverage, and a dash of mindfulness to kickstart your day. Get ready to conquer the world, one sunrise at a time!

Ah, the morning—the gateway to a new day, a fresh start, and endless possibilities. As a mother, your mornings might feel more like chaotic whirlwinds than serene sunrises, but fear not, for we're about to transform your mornings from frenzied to fabulous with a sprinkle of Superconscious Swagger.

First, let's address the elephant in the room: mornings can be tough. Between waking up groggy-eyed, wrangling sleepy kids out of bed, and trying to remember where you left your keys, it's no wonder that mornings often feel like an uphill battle. Here's the secret: by crafting a morning ritual, you can turn even the most chaotic mornings into moments of peace, purpose, and power.

Grab your favorite mug, fill it with your beverage of choice, and dive into the magical world of morning rituals.

The Power of Ritual

Before we dive into the nitty-gritty of crafting your Superconscious morning ritual, let's take a moment to appreciate the power of the word ritual itself. Rituals are more than just habits or routines—they're sacred acts that imbue our lives with meaning, intention, and connection.

Think about it: when you engage in a ritual, whether lighting a candle or simply sipping your morning coffee, you're signaling your brain and spirit that something special is about to happen. Rituals can ground us, center us, and remind us of what truly matters.

That's precisely why crafting a Superconscious morning ritual is so important. By infusing your mornings with intention, mindfulness, and love, you're setting the stage for a day filled with joy, clarity, and purpose.

Designing Your Superconscious Morning Ritual

Now that we understand the power of ritual, let's roll up our sleeves and design a tailor-made morning routine for you. Remember, there's no one-size-fits-all approach to morning rituals—your ritual should reflect your unique preferences, personality, and priorities.

To get started, grab a pen and a journal (or your smartphone, if you prefer digital notetaking) and answer the following questions:

- How do you want to feel when you wake up?

- What routines or habits do you already have in place?

- Are there any new routines or habits you'd like to incorporate?

- How much time can you realistically dedicate to your morning ritual?

- What obstacles or challenges might prevent you from sticking to your ritual, and how can you overcome them?

Once you've answered these questions, it's time to start brainstorming ideas for your Superconscious morning ritual. Here are a few suggestions to get your creative juices flowing:

1. **Mindful Moments:** Start your day with a few minutes of mindfulness meditation or deep breathing. Close your eyes, focus on your breath, and release any tension or stress from the previous day.

2. **Gratitude Practice:** Take a moment to count your blessings and express gratitude for the little things in life. Whether it's a warm cup of coffee, a cozy blanket, or birds chirping outside your window, there's always something to be thankful for.

3. **Set Your Intention for the Day**: You can write down or say aloud how you want your day to unfold. Then, set the intention to do your best to make it happen.

4. **Movement and Exercise:** Get your body moving with gentle stretching, yoga, or a quick workout. Put on a song that motivates you and dance around the kitchen while packing lunches, or maybe add a couple of squats or jumping jacks before showering. Not only will exercise boost your energy levels and mood, but it'll set a positive tone for the rest of your day.

5. **Connection and Communication:** Connect with your loved ones before you go your separate ways for the day. I know that mornings are often a race to get out the door, but take a minute to say something nice to your loved ones; it will make you feel good and help them start their day on a positive note.

6. **Nutritious Nourishment:** Fuel your body with a nutritious breakfast that will nourish your mind, body, and spirit. Whether it's a smoothie packed with fruit and veggies, a hearty bowl of oatmeal, or a simple bowl of yogurt and granola, choose food that makes you feel vibrant and alive. And if breakfast isn't your thing, then pack some veggies or a healthy snack to bring with you.

7. **Nature Connection:** The first time you step outside each day, take a quick look around and soak up the beauty of nature. Breathe in the fresh air and marvel at the wonders of the natural world. Connecting with nature is a powerful way to ground yourself and find inner peace.

Remember, your Superconscious morning routine is yours and yours alone. Feel free to mix and match these ideas, add your personal touches, and experiment until you find a routine that feels right for you.

Putting It into Practice

Now that you've designed your Superconscious morning routine, it's time to put it into practice. Here are a few tips to help you get started:

1. **Start Small:** If you're new to having a conscious morning routine, don't overwhelm yourself by trying to do too much too soon. Start with one or two simple practices and gradually add more as you feel comfortable.

2. **Be Flexible:** Life happens, and sometimes, your morning routine might need to be adjusted or shortened. That's okay! Be flexible and adapt your routine to fit your needs and circumstances.

3. **Stay Consistent:** Consistency is key when it comes to morning routines. Try to stick to your routine as much as possible, even on weekends or holidays. The more consistent you are, the more powerful it will become.

4. **Listen to Your Body:** Pay attention to how your body and mind respond to your morning routine. If something doesn't feel right or isn't serving you, don't be afraid to adjust it or try something new.

5. **Make a List:** Making a list of your morning routine steps and checking each off as you go is a great way to teach your mind to follow through. Practicing something new consistently is the key to shifting your mindset.

6. **Give Yourself Grace:** Remember, your morning routine is meant to support and nourish you, not to stress you out. If you miss a day or don't stick to your routine perfectly, that's okay! Give yourself grace and know that tomorrow is a new day.

Congratulations, you've taken the first step to Superconscious living! You're setting the stage for a day filled with joy, clarity, and purpose by crafting a morning ritual infused with intention, mindfulness, and love. So, pour yourself another cup of coffee (or tea—we're not picky), and get ready to conquer the world, one sunrise at a time.

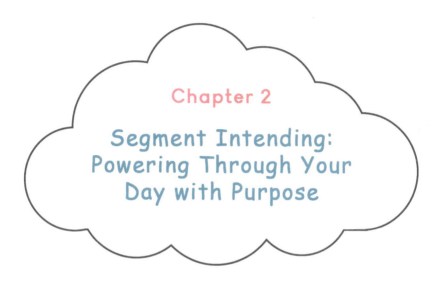

Chapter 2

Segment Intending: Powering Through Your Day with Purpose

Ever feel like your day is a whirlwind of chaos? Well, that's the perfect time to introduce you to the magic of segment intending. Say goodbye to scattered thoughts and hello to focused action! With a sprinkle of Superconscious Swagger, you'll navigate your day like a seasoned captain steering a ship through calm waters.

Welcome to the world of segment intending, an invaluable tool in your Superconscious toolkit for navigating the choppy waters of daily life with grace, clarity, and purpose. In this chapter, we dive deep into the art of segment intending and explore how you can harness its power to transform your days from chaotic to calm, from overwhelming to manageable, and from scattered to focused.

What is Segment Intending?

First, what exactly is segment intending, and how does it differ from traditional goal-setting or time-management techniques? At its core, segment intending is about breaking your day into smaller, manageable segments and setting clear intentions for each segment.

Imagine your day as a series of chapters in a book, each with its own unique theme, setting, and cast of characters. With segment intending, you become the author of your story, consciously choosing the direction you want each chapter of your day to take and infusing it with intention, purpose, and meaning.

The Benefits of Segment Intending

So, why bother with segment intending? What are the benefits of breaking your day into bite-sized chunks and setting intentions for each segment? The answer lies in the power of focus, clarity, and momentum.

When you set clear intentions for each segment of your day, you eliminate the guesswork and indecision that often lead to procrastinating, feeling overwhelmed, and burning out. Instead of feeling at the mercy of external forces, you become the master of your destiny, confidently charting a course toward your goals and dreams.

Segment intending also helps you stay present and engaged, fully immersing yourself in whatever task or activity you're focused on without being distracted by thoughts of past or future obligations.

You will maximize your productivity, creativity, and overall fulfillment by bringing your full attention and energy to each segment of your day.

Powering Through Your Day with Purpose

Now that we understand the what and why of segment intending, let's dive into the how. How can you incorporate segment intending into your daily routine, and what are some practical tips for making the most of this powerful technique? Here are a few strategies to get you started:

1. **Set Clear Intentions:** Before you begin each segment of your day, take a moment to pause, breathe, and set a clear intention for what you want to accomplish. Whether completing a project, having a productive meeting, or simply enjoying a moment of relaxation, be intentional about how you want to show up in each segment of your day.

2. **Prioritize Your Tasks:** Not all segments of your day are created equal. Some may be more important or time-sensitive than others, so prioritize your tasks and activities accordingly. List the most important tasks you must accomplish daily and allocate your time and energy accordingly.

3. **Stay Flexible:** While setting intentions is important, staying flexible and adaptable as the day unfolds is also important. Life has a way of throwing curveballs when we least expect it, so be prepared to adjust your plans and intentions as needed. Remember, it's not about being rigid or controlling—it's about staying focused and intentional in uncertainty.

4. **Practice Mindfulness:** Mindfulness is the key to successful segment intending. Stay present and engaged in each segment of your day, bringing your full attention and awareness to whatever task or activity you focus on. Resist the temptation to

multitask or let your mind wander to past or future obligations and stay grounded in the here and now.

5. **Giving Dreaded Tasks Purpose:** When faced with tasks you dread doing, using segment intending as positive thoughts and prayers for those in need can be especially powerful. For example, before tackling your dreaded task, set an intention to offer up the completion of your task as a positive vibe or prayer for someone who could use your love and support. I have done this many times with an entire day of work by using each hour as a separate intention for someone I knew needed help or by sending it out as love into the universe to the people who need it most.

Putting It into Practice

Now that you have a solid understanding of segment intending and some tips for incorporating it into your daily routine, it's time to put it into practice. Here's a step-by-step guide to help you get started:

1. **Map Out Your Day:** Start by mapping out your day into segments, considering any recurring commitments, appointments, or obligations you have. Divide your day into chunks of time that make sense, whether by the hour, task, or activity.

2. **Set Intentions:** Before you begin each segment of your day, take a moment to set a clear intention for what you want to accomplish. Write it down if it helps, or simply hold it in your mind and heart as you go about your day.

3. **Stay Present:** As you move through each segment of your day, stay present and engaged in the moment. Focus on whatever task or activity you're doing and resist the temptation to multitask or let your mind wander.

4. **Adjust as Needed:** Be prepared to adjust your plans and intentions as needed as the day unfolds. Life is full of unexpected twists and turns, so stay flexible and adaptable in the face of uncertainty.

5. **Reflect and Review:** At the end of each segment or at the end of each day, take a few moments to reflect on how things went. Celebrate your successes, learn from any challenges or setbacks, and use this feedback to adjust your intentions and strategies moving forward.

Congratulations, you've unlocked the power of segment intending! By breaking your day into manageable segments and setting clear intentions for each, you're empowering yourself to navigate life with purpose, focus, and grace. So, embrace the magic of segment intending, and watch as your days unfold with clarity and purpose!

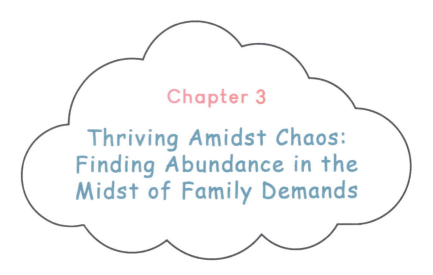

Chapter 3

**Thriving Amidst Chaos:
Finding Abundance in the
Midst of Family Demands**

Are you overwhelmed by the demands of raising a
family, juggling multiple activities, and struggling to
keep up with financial obligations? In this chapter, we
delve into practical strategies for shifting your mindset about debt and scarcity and embracing a mindset
of abundance, even amidst chaos.

As a busy mom with kids engaged in multiple sports and activities, it's easy to get caught up in the whirlwind of daily life and feel overwhelmed by financial pressures. The constant juggling of bills and expenses and trying to keep up with the seemingly perfect lives portrayed on social media can take a toll on your mental and emotional well-being. However, it's essential to recognize that abundance is not just about material wealth; it's about cultivating a mindset of gratitude, resourcefulness, and resilience that will allow you to thrive, regardless of your circumstances.

Thriving Amidst Chaos

So, how do you shift your mindset about debt and scarcity and embrace a mindset of abundance, even amidst chaos? Here are two strategies you can begin using:

1. **Gratitude Practice**: Take a moment each day to acknowledge the abundance in your life, whether it's the love of your family, the roof over your head, or the simple pleasures of everyday life like the smell of freshly brewed coffee. Cultivating an attitude of gratitude can help shift your focus away from scarcity and toward abundance, reminding you of the richness and blessings surrounding you.

2. **Focus on Solutions, Not Problems**: Instead of dwelling on your financial challenges, focus on finding solutions and taking proactive steps to improve your situation. Whether creating a budget, cutting unnecessary expenses, or exploring additional income opportunities, adopting a solutions mindset can help you feel more empowered and in control of your finances.

Putting It into Practice

Now that you have a couple of strategies for an abundant mindset, here are two practices to get you started:

1. **Create a Financial Vision Board**: Visualize your financial goals by creating a vision board representing your ideal financial future. Include images and words that inspire and motivate you, such as pictures of your dream home, vacation destinations, or financial milestones. Display your vision board in a place where you can see it daily as a constant reminder of what you're working toward.

2. **Practice Abundance Mentality**: Cultivate an abundance mindset by shifting your perspective on money and wealth. Instead of viewing money as the ultimate measure of success or happiness, recognize it as a tool that allows you to acquire the things you value. Understand that money isn't inherently powerful itself—it's simply a means of exchange that gives you more choices and opportunities to pursue what brings you joy and fulfillment. Focus on gratitude for the resources you already have and the abundance that surrounds you, whether it's the love of your family, the beauty of nature, or the experiences that enrich your life. Reframing your relationship with money and wealth can cultivate a sense of abundance beyond your bank account. Surround yourself with positive influences, such as supportive friends and family members, who will reinforce this perspective and inspire you to embrace abundance in all areas of your life.

Remember that true abundance is not measured by the size of your bank account or the possessions you own but by the richness of your relationships, the depth of your experiences, and the joy and fulfillment you find in everyday life. By shifting your mindset about debt and scarcity and embracing a mindset of abundance, you can reclaim control of your finances and create a life of prosperity and fulfillment for you and your family, even amidst the chaos of daily routines.

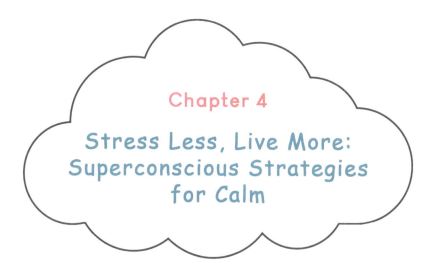

Chapter 4

Stress Less, Live More: Superconscious Strategies for Calm

Stress? Busy moms don't have time for that! Learn how to kick stress to the curb with our Superconscious strategies. From laughter therapy to guided visualization, we've got the tools to help you reclaim your Zen like a boss. So, take a deep breath, exhale the stress, and let's dive in!

Let's talk about what it means to stress less and live more. In this chapter, we embark on a journey to banish stress from our lives using the power of Superconscious strategies. Stress may be a familiar companion in our hectic lives, but with the right tools and techniques, we can kick it to the curb and reclaim our peace, joy, and vitality.

Understanding Stress

Before diving into stress management strategies, let's take a minute to understand what it is and how it affects us. Stress is the body's natural response to perceived threats or challenges, triggering a cascade of physiological and psychological responses designed to help us cope with danger.

Stress can be beneficial in small doses, helping us stay focused, motivated, and alert when facing challenges. However, when stress becomes overwhelming, it can have serious consequences for our physical, mental, and emotional health and contribute to a wide range of health problems, including heart disease, anxiety, depression, and more.

The Superconscious Approach to Stress Management

So, how can we manage stress in a way that honors our minds, bodies, and spirits? Enter the Superconscious approach to stress management, a holistic, integrative approach that combines cutting-edge science with ancient wisdom to help us reclaim our peace, joy, and vitality.

At its core, the Superconscious approach to stress management is about tapping into the power of our Superconscious minds—the part of our consciousness that transcends the limitations of our egos and connects us to a higher source of wisdom, guidance, and healing. By harnessing the power of our Superconscious minds, we can access deep reservoirs of inner peace, resilience, and well-being that allow us to navigate life's challenges gracefully and easily.

Superconscious Strategies for Stress Management

Now that we understand the Superconscious approach to stress management, let's explore some practical strategies for banishing stress from our lives and reclaiming our peace, joy, and vitality. Here are a few Superconscious strategies to get you started:

1. **Laughter Therapy:** Laughter is the best stress management medicine. Not only does laughter release feel-good endorphins and reduce levels of stress hormones in the body, but it also helps us shift our perspectives and find humor in even the most challenging situations. So, go ahead, my friends—watch a funny movie, tell a joke, or simply laugh at yourself and let the stress melt away.

2. **Guided Visualization:** Guided visualization is a powerful tool for reducing stress and promoting relaxation. By closing your eyes and imagining yourself in a peaceful, serene environment—a lush forest, a tranquil beach, or a cozy mountain cabin—you can create a sense of calm and tranquility that will soothe your body, mind, and spirit. So, find a quiet space, close your eyes, and let your imagination take you on a journey to inner peace.

3. **Mindful Movement:** Movement is a powerful antidote to stress, helping to release tension from the body and calm the mind. Whether it's yoga, tai chi, walking in nature, or putting on your favorite song and having an impromptu dance party in your living room, find a form of movement that brings you joy and helps you connect with your body and breath. Practice mindfulness as you move, focusing your attention on the movement of your body and the rhythm of your breath, and let the stress melt away with every step.

4. **Breathwork:** Deep breathing is one of the simplest and most effective ways to reduce stress and promote relaxation. By slowing down your breath and taking long, deep breaths into your belly, you activate the body's relaxation response, triggering a cascade of physiological changes that promote calmness and well-being. Practice deep breathing throughout the day whenever you feel stressed or overwhelmed and feel the tension melt away with each breath.

5. **De-Stress Countdown:** One of the easiest and most effective techniques is combining breathwork with counting. Take a slow, deep breath through your nose, hold it for a few seconds, count one, two, three, then slowly blow it out through your mouth, counting backward from three, two, one.

6. **Self-Compassion:** Finally, practice self-compassion as you navigate the ups and downs of life. Be kind and gentle with yourself, especially during times of stress and difficulty, and remember that it's okay to ask for help and support when needed. Treat yourself with the same love, care, and understanding you would offer to a dear friend, and watch as your stress melts away in the warm embrace of self-compassion.

Putting It into Practice

Now that you have a toolbox full of Superconscious strategies for managing stress, it's time to put them into practice. Here's a step-by-step guide to help you banish stress from your life and reclaim your peace, joy, and vitality:

1. **Identify Your Stress Triggers:** Start by identifying the sources of stress in your life—the people, situations, and circumstances that trigger feelings of stress and anxiety. Once

you've identified your stress triggers, you can develop strategies for managing them more effectively.

2. **Practice Self-Awareness:** Pay attention to your thoughts, feelings, and physical sensations throughout the day, especially when experiencing stress. Notice any patterns or tendencies that arise, and practice self-awareness and self-compassion as you navigate the ups and downs of life.

3. **Choose Your Superconscious Strategies:** Choose one or more Superconscious strategies from the list above—or any other techniques that resonate with you—and incorporate them into your daily routine. Experiment with different strategies to see what works best for you, and don't be afraid to mix and match until you find the perfect combination for managing stress.

4. **Stay Consistent:** Consistency is key when managing stress. Commit to practicing your chosen Superconscious strategies regularly to build resilience and cultivate inner peace and well-being even when you're not stressed.

5. **Seek Support:** Finally, don't be afraid to seek support from friends, family, or professional counselors if you struggle to manage stress alone. Remember, you don't have to go it alone—there's strength in reaching out for help and support when you need it most.

Congratulations, amazing moms—you've unlocked the power of Superconscious stress management! By incorporating laughter therapy, guided visualization, mindful movement, breathwork, and self-compassion into your daily routine, you're reclaiming your peace, joy, and vitality one Superconscious strategy at a time. So, kick stress to the curb like a boss and embrace the calm, centered, and empowered version of yourself that's waiting to emerge!

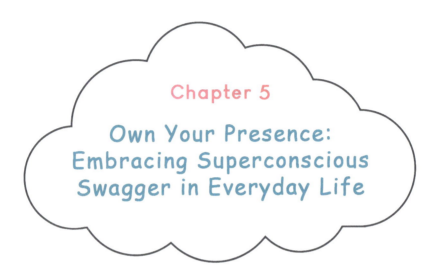

Chapter 5

Own Your Presence:
Embracing Superconscious
Swagger in Everyday Life

Step into the realm of transformation, where confidence meets intentionality. In this chapter, we'll delve into the art of infusing your daily existence with Superconscious Swagger, whether you're at home, at work, or cheering on your kids from the sidelines. Picture this: every interaction, every decision, every moment —imbued with a sense of purpose and self-assurance. Get ready to elevate your life to new heights, one empowered step at a time!

Ah, the intricate steps of juggling responsibilities, navigating challenges, and embracing moments of joy. As a mom, you've likely mastered the art of multitasking and resilience, yet amid the hustle and bustle, it's easy to lose sight of your own power and presence. That's where Superconscious Swagger comes in—a potent blend of confidence, mindfulness, and authenticity that will propel you forward with grace and determination.

Igniting Confidence with Superconscious Strategies

So, now you understand the importance of infusing your daily existence with Superconscious Swagger. Below are a few strategies to own your power and presence with confidence in everyday life:

1. **Living Space Mastery**: Transform your home into a confident sanctuary by decluttering and organizing with intention. Designate spaces for morning rituals and evening relaxation to cultivate calm and clarity.

2. **Appearance Empowerment**: Boost your confidence by pampering yourself with a simple yet luxurious beauty routine. Looking and feeling good will help you radiate confidence.

3. **Workday Command**: Shine confidently in the workplace by cultivating a positive, professional mindset. Set clear goals, establish boundaries, and embrace challenges as opportunities for growth. Leverage your strengths to overcome obstacles and propel yourself to success.

4. **Event Cheerleading**: Be your child's biggest supporter at sporting events and extracurricular activities by shifting your perspective from spectator to cheerleader. Celebrate their journey with enthusiasm and pride and foster a supportive community with like-minded moms.

Putting It into Practice

Now that you know a few strategies to build your confidence, here are four practices to help you get started:

1. **Own Your Living Space Like a Boss:** Your home is your sanctuary, reflecting your values and aspirations. Infuse each room intentionally, from your morning routine to your evening wind-down. Clear out the clutter to promote clarity of mind and peace of spirit.

2. **Looking the Part**: Before entering the world, take a minute to ignite your confidence through personal hygiene and appearance. Create a simple yet indulgent beauty routine. Take a cleansing shower, blow out your hair, or style it to perfection, swipe on a coat of mascara, and spritz on a scent that uplifts your mood and invigorates your senses. You might be empowered to adorn yourself with a special piece of jewelry that symbolizes confidence when you wear it, then slip into your designer shoes or favorite sneakers—whatever makes you feel like the radiant mom you are. When you put a little effort into looking and feeling good, you exude confidence effortlessly.

3. **Strutting Through Your Workday:** Command Your domain. Whether you're climbing the corporate ladder or pursuing your passion project, let your Superconscious Swagger shine in the workplace. Cultivate a confident mindset that exudes professionalism and poise. Whenever you catch yourself amidst negative self-talk, pause and reframe your thoughts. Replace self-criticism with words of encouragement and affirmation. Stand tall, with your shoulders back and your chin up. Stay away from office drama and make a conscious effort to connect with others through eye contact and attentiveness. Set clear goals and boundaries, prioritize tasks with precision and purpose, only take on what you can handle, and delegate when

necessary. Embrace challenges as opportunities for growth, leveraging your strengths to overcome obstacles with finesse.

4. **Cheerleading at Events:** Seeing your children grow and flourish through sports and activities is a source of immeasurable pride and joy. Although the sidelines can often be a breeding ground for self-doubt and comparison, choose not to participate. Shift your perspective from spectator to cheerleader, celebrating your child's journey with unwavering support and enthusiasm. They may not play well every game, but knowing you are proud of them regardless helps them build their confidence. So, connect with fellow like-minded moms and foster a sense of camaraderie and community that will uplift and inspire your children.

Congratulations on embarking upon this journey of self-discovery and empowerment, my friends. By embracing Superconscious Swagger in every facet of your life, you're reclaiming your inherent worth and embracing your full potential. So, stand tall, speak your truth, and navigate life's twists and turns with unwavering confidence. The world is yours to conquer, one empowered moment at a time!

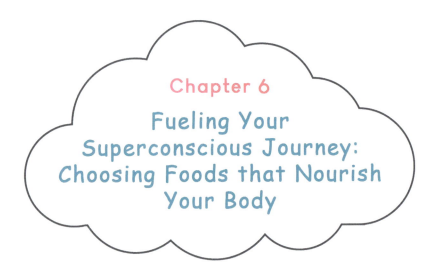

Chapter 6

Fueling Your Superconscious Journey: Choosing Foods that Nourish Your Body

Welcome to the next stage of your Superconscious journey, where we dive into the vital importance of nourishing your body and mind for optimal performance. Just like a superhero needs the proper fuel to save the day, you need the right nutrients to power through your daily adventures with Superconscious Swagger. Get ready to fuel your body, ignite your mind, and conquer the world, one healthy choice at a time!

In today's fast-paced world, it's easy to neglect our bodies and minds in favor of convenience and instant gratification, but just as a car needs premium fuel to run smoothly, your body and mind require proper nourishment to function at their best. By prioritizing healthy eating habits throughout the day, you can supercharge your energy levels, boost your mood, and unleash your full potential with Superconscious Swagger.

Fueling Your Superconscious Journey

Below are four tips to begin nourishing your body and mind for optimal performance:

1. **Start Strong with Superconscious Breakfasts**: Kickstart your day with a nutritious breakfast that will set the tone for success. Instead of reaching for sugary cereals or carb-heavy pastries, opt for whole foods that provide sustained energy and mental clarity. Think oatmeal topped with fresh berries and nuts, avocado toast with tomato, or a protein-packed smoothie filled with leafy greens and antioxidant-rich fruits. By fueling your body with wholesome ingredients, you'll feel energized and empowered to tackle whatever the day throws your way.

2. **Stay Energized with Smart Snacking**: When hunger strikes between meals, reach for snacks that nourish your body and stabilize your energy levels. Stock up on portable options like fresh fruit, nuts, seeds, and protein bars for quick and easy fuel on the go. Instead of reaching for sugary or processed snacks that leave you feeling sluggish and unsatisfied, choose whole foods that provide sustained energy and mental focus. With smart snacking, you'll stay energized and alert throughout the day, ready to tackle any challenge confidently and clearly.

3. **Power Up Your Lunch and Dinner**: Make mealtime a celebration of nourishment and flavor by incorporating nutrient-dense ingredients into your lunch and dinner menus.

Load up on colorful vegetables, lean proteins, whole grains, and healthy fats to fuel your body with the ingredients it needs to thrive. Experiment with new recipes and flavors to keep your meals exciting and satisfying. Don't forget to listen to your body's hunger and fullness cues to ensure you're eating mindfully and intuitively. With a balanced and varied diet, you'll be nourished from the inside out, ready to take on whatever life throws your way.

4. **Satisfy Nighttime Cravings with Healthy Alternatives**: Instead of reaching for sugary desserts or salty snacks late at night, satisfy your cravings with healthy alternatives that will nourish your body and support restful sleep. Opt for a bowl of Greek yogurt with fresh fruit and a drizzle of honey, a handful of mixed nuts and seeds, or a piece of dark chocolate paired with herbal tea. If you find yourself mindlessly snacking while watching TV or scrolling through your phone, try chewing mint gum or brushing your teeth after your last snack to signal to your brain that eating time is over. With these healthy nighttime habits, you'll support your body's natural rhythms and wake up feeling refreshed and rejuvenated, ready to tackle a new day with Superconscious Swagger.

Incorporate these practices into your daily routine, and watch as you fuel your body and mind for success with Superconscious Swagger. Remember, you have the power to nourish yourself from the inside out and unleash your full potential in every aspect of your life. So, go ahead, my friends—fuel up and conquer the world with confidence and vitality!

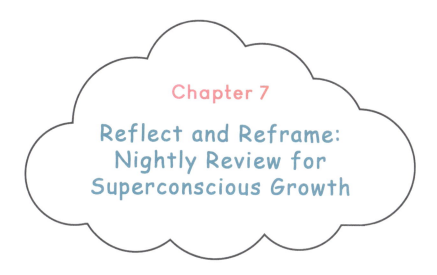

Chapter 7

Reflect and Reframe: Nightly Review for Superconscious Growth

Lights, camera, reflection! Join us as we roll the tape on your day and uncover the hidden gems of wisdom waiting to be discovered. With a dash of Superconscious Swagger, you'll learn to reframe challenges as opportunities and transform setbacks into stepping-stones toward your dreams.

Welcome, my friends, to reflect and reframe—a nightly review for Superconscious growth. In this chapter, we delve into the transformative power of reflection, showing you how to review your day with a discerning eye and reframe your experiences through the lens of Superconscious Swagger. So, grab your popcorn and settle in as we embark on a journey of self-discovery and growth.

The Importance of Reflection

Before we dive into the practical strategies for nightly reflection, let's take a moment to explore why reflection is such a crucial component of personal growth and development. Reflection is more than just a passive recounting of events—it's an active process of self-awareness and introspection that allows us to learn from our experiences, identify patterns and themes, and gain valuable insights into ourselves and our lives.

By reflecting on our day, we can gain clarity about our thoughts, feelings, and actions, uncovering hidden motivations, beliefs, and desires that may be driving our behavior. Reflection also allows us to celebrate our successes, acknowledge our challenges, and identify areas for growth and improvement, empowering us to make conscious choices and take intentional action toward our goals and dreams.

The Nightly Review Process

So, how can we cultivate a nightly review practice that fosters Superconscious growth and development? Fortunately, there are countless ways to approach nightly reflection; all it takes is a willingness to set aside a little time each evening to review your day with intention and curiosity. Here's a simple yet powerful process to get you started:

1. **Set the Scene:** Find a quiet, comfortable space to sit or lie down without distractions. Dim the lights, light a candle,

or play soft music to create a calm and peaceful atmosphere conducive to reflection.

2. **Review Your Day:** Begin by mentally reviewing your day from start to finish, recalling the events, interactions, and experiences that occurred. Take a few moments to acknowledge and honor the highs and lows of your day, allowing yourself to fully experience and process your emotions.

3. **Identify Successes:** Next, identify and celebrate the successes and accomplishments of your day, no matter how small or seemingly insignificant. Perhaps you completed a challenging task, made progress toward a goal, or shared a meaningful connection with a loved one. Whatever it may be, take a moment to savor the pride, satisfaction, and joy accompanying your achievements.

4. **Acknowledge Challenges:** Similarly, acknowledge and honor the challenges and difficulties you encountered throughout your day. Perhaps you've faced obstacles, setbacks, or disappointments that tested your resilience and resolve. Instead of dwelling on the negative, view these challenges as opportunities for growth and learning, recognizing the lessons and insights they offer.

5. **Reframe Perspectives:** With a spirit of Superconscious Swagger, reframe your perspectives on the challenges, setbacks, and disappointments, seeing them as valuable opportunities for growth, learning, and transformation. Ask yourself: What can I learn from this experience? How can I grow stronger, wiser, and more resilient? By reframing challenges in this way, you'll cultivate a mindset of optimism, resilience, and empowerment that will propel you forward on your journey of Superconscious growth.

Putting It into Practice

Now that you understand the nightly review process, it's time to put it into practice. Here's a step-by-step guide to help you cultivate a nightly review practice that will foster Superconscious growth and development:

1. **Set Aside Time:** Set aside dedicated time each evening to engage in your nightly review practice before bedtime or after dinner. Set aside five to ten minutes for this activity. Make it a non-negotiable part of your day, prioritizing your growth and well-being.

2. **Create a Routine:** Create a routine or ritual around your nightly review practice to make it feel special and sacred. Light a candle, brew a cup of tea, or journal in a cozy blanket— whatever helps you feel grounded, centered, and present in the moment.

3. **Start Small:** Begin by focusing on one or two aspects of your day you'd like to review and reflect on, such as your interactions with others, your progress toward your goals, or your self-care practices. Start small and gradually expand your focus over time as you become more comfortable with the process.

4. **Be Honest and Authentic:** Approach your nightly review practice with honesty, authenticity, and self-compassion, allowing yourself to fully experience and express your thoughts, feelings, and emotions. Be gentle with yourself, recognizing that growth and learning are ongoing processes that require patience, persistence, and self-love.

5. **Celebrate Your Progress:** Finally, celebrate your progress and growth, acknowledging the insights, lessons, and breakthroughs that emerge through your nightly reflection practice. Celebrate the small victories, honor the challenges, and embrace the journey of self-discovery and growth with open arms.

The Power of Personal Growth

As you cultivate a nightly review practice, you'll discover a newfound sense of clarity, purpose, and empowerment that will propel you forward on your journey of personal growth and transformation. You'll learn to reframe challenges as opportunities, transform setbacks into steppingstones, and embrace the limitless possibilities that await you with each new day.

Congratulations, you've unlocked the power of nightly reflection! By embracing the nightly review process and infusing it with Superconscious Swagger, you're cultivating a growth, resilience, and empowerment mindset that propels you forward on your journey of self-discovery and transformation. So, go ahead, ladies—roll the tape on your day, reflect on your experiences, and reframe your perspectives with a dash of Superconscious Swagger.

PART 2

Radiate Your Connections: Superconscious Strategies for Relationships

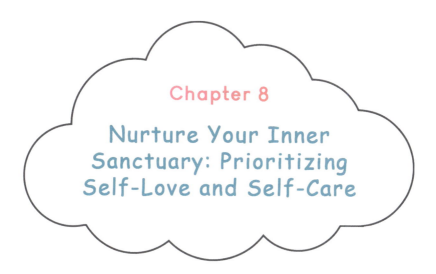

Chapter 8

Nurture Your Inner Sanctuary: Prioritizing Self-Love and Self-Care

Time to pamper your most important VIP: yourself! In this chapter, we dive into the art of self-love and create a sanctuary of Superconscious self-care. From bubble baths (or hot showers!) to boundary-setting, we'll explore how to nourish your mind, body, and spirit like the goddess (or superhero) you are.

Say hello to the self-love sanctuary, a journey into the depths of self-care and the transformative power of self-love. In a world that often glorifies busyness and self-sacrifice, prioritizing self-care can feel like an act of rebellion, a declaration that your well-being matters just as much as anyone else's. So, grab your favorite scented candles, slip into your coziest pj's, and embark on a journey of self-discovery, healing, and empowerment.

The Importance of Self-Love

Before we dive into the practical strategies for cultivating a self-love sanctuary, let's take a moment to explore why self-love is such a crucial component of well-being and personal growth. Self-love is more than just a warm fuzzy feeling—it's an act of self-acceptance, self-compassion, and self-respect that honors your inherent worth and dignity as a human being.

When prioritizing self-love, we honor our needs, desires, and boundaries, creating greater happiness, fulfillment, and authenticity. Self-love also serves as a foundation for healthy relationships, allowing us to show up as our truest selves and connect with others from a place of wholeness and integrity.

Creating Your Self-Love Sanctuary

So, how can we cultivate a self-love sanctuary, a sacred space dedicated to nourishing our minds, bodies, and spirits with love, care, and compassion? Fortunately, my fellow moms, there are countless ways to create a self-love sanctuary; all it takes is a willingness to prioritize your well-being and make self-care a non-negotiable part of your daily routine. Here are a few simple yet powerful strategies to get you started:

1. **Set Boundaries:** Begin by setting clear and healthy boundaries in your life with yourself and others. Learn to say no to activities, commitments, and relationships that drain your

energy or compromise your well-being, and prioritize activities, commitments, and relationships that nourish and uplift you.

2. **Practice Self-Compassion:** Cultivate a practice of self-compassion by treating yourself with kindness, understanding, and patience, especially during times of difficulty or challenge. Instead of criticizing yourself for perceived flaws or shortcomings, offer yourself the same love and compassion you would offer a dear friend.

3. **Nourish Your Body:** Take care of your physical health by nourishing your body with nutritious food, regular exercise, and plenty of rest and relaxation. Pay attention to your body's signals and needs and honor them with love and care, knowing that your body is your sacred vessel for experiencing life.

4. **Feed Your Mind:** Nourish your mind with uplifting and inspiring content that feeds your soul and expands your consciousness. Whether reading a book, listening to a podcast, or attending a workshop, seek opportunities for growth, learning, and self-discovery that resonate with your interests and values.

5. **Cultivate Joy:** Prioritize activities and experiences that bring you joy, pleasure, and fulfillment, whether in nature, pursuing creative hobbies, or connecting with loved ones. Embrace life's simple pleasures and savor each moment with gratitude and appreciation.

Putting It into Practice

Now that you understand the importance of self-love and have some strategies for creating your self-love sanctuary, it's time to put it into practice. Here's a step-by-step guide to help you cultivate a practice of self-love and self-care that will nourish your mind, body, and spirit:

1. **Create A Sacred Space:** Create a physical space in your home that will serve as your self-love sanctuary, a place where you can retreat and recharge in times of need. Fill this space with objects, images, and scents that bring you joy and comfort, and make it a regular part of your daily routine to spend time there engaging in self-care activities. If space is limited, choose a comfortable chair you can call dibs on for an allotted amount of time each day.

2. **Set Daily Intentions:** Start each day by setting intentions for how you want to prioritize self-love and self-care in your life. Write down one or two self-care activities or practices you will commit to each day, whether it's taking a relaxing bath or a long shower, going for a walk in nature, practicing mindfulness meditation, reading a book, or listening to a podcast or your favorite music.

3. **Practice Mindful Self-Compassion:** Throughout the day, practice mindful self-compassion by tuning into your thoughts, feelings, and sensations with curiosity and kindness. Notice any self-critical or judgmental thoughts and gently reframe them with words of love and encouragement.

4. **Connect with Other Like-Minded Moms:** Remember that self-love and self-care are not selfish acts; they're essential practices that allow you to show up as your best self and contribute positively to the world around you. Connect with others who share your values and interests and support each other on your journey of self-discovery and growth.

The Power of Superconscious Self-Love

As you cultivate a self-love sanctuary infused with Superconscious Swagger, you'll discover a newfound sense of wholeness, authenticity, and empowerment that will transform every aspect of your life. You'll learn to honor your needs, desires, and boundaries with love and respect and create a life that reflects your truest values and aspirations.

So, go ahead—pamper yourself like the VIP you are, and create a self-love sanctuary that will nourish your mind, body, and spirit with love, care, and compassion. With each act of self-love, you'll plant seeds of growth, healing, and transformation that will blossom and flourish in the garden of your heart, enriching your life with beauty, joy, and abundance.

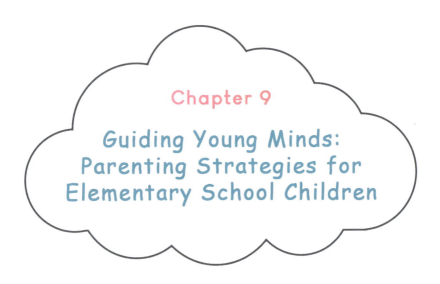

Chapter 9

Guiding Young Minds: Parenting Strategies for Elementary School Children

Welcome to a chapter dedicated to nurturing the budding minds of elementary school children with Superconscious Swagger. This chapter will explore positive parenting strategies to foster growth, confidence, and resilience in your young ones. From fostering independence to setting clear expectations, get ready to empower your children to thrive with Superconscious Swagger.

Parenting elementary school children is a journey of wonder, discovery, and growth. As your child explores the world around them and begins to assert their independence, it's essential to provide guidance and support while nurturing their natural curiosity and creativity.

Guiding Young Minds

Below are five positive parenting strategies to help you navigate the elementary school years with Superconscious Swagger:

1. **Encourage Independence**: Foster your child's sense of autonomy by encouraging them to take on age-appropriate responsibilities and make decisions for themselves. Offer praise and encouragement when they demonstrate independence and resist the urge to intervene unless necessary. By empowering your child to take ownership of their actions and choices, you'll help them develop confidence and self-reliance.

2. **Practice Positive Reinforcement**: Focus on highlighting and praising your child's strengths and achievements rather than dwelling on mistakes or shortcomings. Offer specific, sincere praise for their efforts and accomplishments and celebrate their successes, whether big or small. By focusing on positivity and encouragement, you help your child develop a growth mindset and resilience in the face of challenges.

3. **Set Clear Expectations**: Establish clear, consistent expectations for your child's behavior and responsibilities, and communicate them positively and neutrally. Be firm but fair when enforcing rules and consequences, and explain the reasons behind your expectations. Setting clear boundaries provides structure and stability for your child while teaching them valuable lessons about accountability and respect.

4. **Foster Open Communication**: Create a safe, supportive environment where your child will feel comfortable expressing

their thoughts, feelings, and concerns. Listen actively and attentively when your child speaks and validate their emotions without judgment. Encourage open dialogue and honest communication, and be willing to address any questions or concerns your child may have. By fostering a culture of open communication, you'll strengthen your bond with your child and build trust and mutual respect.

5. **Lead by Example**: Be a positive role model for your child by demonstrating kindness, empathy, and integrity in your words and actions. Treat others with respect and compassion and strive to resolve conflicts peacefully and constructively. Show your child the importance of honesty, responsibility, and perseverance through your behavior, and encourage them to emulate these values in their lives. By leading by example, you'll instill important moral and ethical principles in your child and empower them to become compassionate individuals.

Putting It into Practice

Now that you have a solid foundation of how to guide young minds with positive parenting strategies, it's time to put them into practice:

1. **Encourage Independence:** Encourage your child to take on new responsibilities at home, such as helping with chores or making their own lunch.

2. **Practice Positive Reinforcement:** Take time each day to praise your child for their efforts and accomplishments and celebrate their successes together as a family.

3. **Set Clear Expectations:** Sit down with your child, discuss your family's rules and expectations, and collaborate on creating a set of guidelines everyone can agree upon.

4. **Foster Open Communication:** Schedule regular family meetings where everyone can share their thoughts, feelings, and ideas in a safe and supportive environment.

5. **Lead by Example:** Model positive communication skills and behavior in interactions with your child and others.

By implementing these strategies into your parenting approach, you can empower your child to thrive academically, socially, and emotionally, setting them up for success in school and beyond. So, go ahead—buckle up and get ready to guide your young ones through the exciting elementary school journey with confidence, compassion, and Superconscious Swagger!

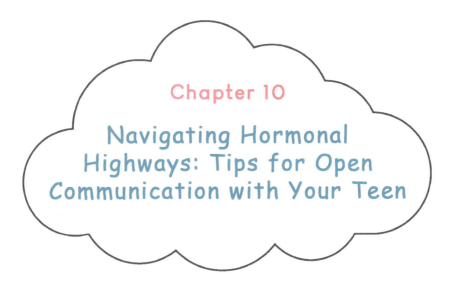

Chapter 10

Navigating Hormonal Highways: Tips for Open Communication with Your Teen

Welcome to a chapter dedicated to navigating the choppy waters of communication with your teens during their hormone-fueled journey through adolescence. This chapter will explore tips, strategies, and Superconscious techniques for fostering open, honest, and meaningful communication with your teens. From active listening to setting boundaries, strengthen your parent-teen bond with a Superconscious approach.

Welcome to a chapter dedicated to navigating the hormonal highways of adolescence with open communication, empathy, and Superconscious awareness. This chapter will explore the challenges and complexities of parenting teens undergoing hormonal changes and share practical tips for fostering healthy communication and connection.

Parenting a teenager can feel like navigating uncharted territory filled with twists, turns, and unexpected detours. As your teen experiences hormonal changes and grapples with newfound independence, it's essential to maintain an open line of communication and cultivate a supportive, trusting relationship.

Navigating Hormonal Highways

Effective communication is the key to navigating the hormonal highways of adolescence with grace and understanding. By fostering open, honest dialogue with your teen, you can strengthen your bond, build mutual respect, and navigate challenges together as a team. Below are five strategies to get you started:

1. **Listen With Empathy**: When your teen comes to you with a problem or concern, listen empathetically and without judgment. Validate their feelings and tell them you're there to support them, no matter what. Avoid interrupting or jumping to conclusions; give them the space to express themselves fully and openly.

2. **Be Present and Engaged**: Put down your phone, turn off the TV, and give your teen your full attention when they're talking to you. Make eye contact, nod your head, and use active listening techniques to show you are fully engaged in the conversation. Being present and attentive demonstrates that you value their thoughts and feelings.

3. **Set Boundaries with Compassion**: While giving your teen space to express themselves is important, setting clear

boundaries and expectations is also crucial. Be firm but compassionate when enforcing rules and consequences, and explain the reasons behind your decisions. By setting boundaries with love and understanding, you'll help your teens feel safe and supported as they navigate the challenges of adolescence.

4. **Create Opportunities for Connection**: Find activities or hobbies that you and your teen can enjoy together. Use these shared experiences as opportunities to bond and connect more deeply. Spending quality time together will strengthen your relationship and create lasting memories.

Practice Patience and Understanding

Parenting a teenager can be challenging, but it's essential to practice patience and understanding, even when tensions run high. Remember that your teen is going through intense growth and change, both physically and emotionally. Approach conflicts with empathy and compassion and strive to see things from their perspective.

Putting It into Practice

Now that you have strategies for how to navigate your teen's hormonal highways, it's time to put them into practice:

1. **Listen with Empathy:** When your teen opens up about a problem or concern, resist the urge to jump in with advice or judgment. Instead, listen empathetically, validating their emotions and reassuring them of your support. Let them know it's okay to express themselves fully, without fear of criticism or interruption. Practice active listening by paraphrasing their words and reflecting back their feelings, showing genuine understanding and empathy.

2. **Be Present and Engaged:** Show your teen they have your undivided attention by putting away distractions like your

phone or pausing the TV. Make eye contact, nod your head, and use nonverbal cues to convey that you're fully present and engaged in the conversation. By eliminating distractions and focusing solely on your teen, you will demonstrate respect for their thoughts and feelings, fostering a deeper sense of connection and trust.

3. **Set Boundaries with Compassion:** While it's important to be understanding and supportive, it's equally important to establish clear boundaries and expectations. Approach rule-setting with empathy and compassion, explaining the reasons behind your decisions and enforcing consequences with love and understanding. By setting boundaries rooted in compassion, you will provide your teen with structure and guidance while respecting their autonomy and individuality.

4. **Create Opportunities for Connection:** Strengthen your bond with your teen by finding activities or hobbies you can enjoy together. Whether it's cooking a meal, going for a walk, or watching a movie, shared experiences provide valuable opportunities for bonding and connection. Use these moments to engage in meaningful conversation and build memories that will last a lifetime.

5. **Practice Patience and Understanding:** Parenting a teenager requires a hefty dose of patience and understanding, especially during moments of conflict or tension. Keep in mind that your teen is navigating a period of intense growth and change, both physically and emotionally. Approach challenges with empathy and compassion, striving to see things from their perspective and validating their feelings even when you disagree. By modeling patience and understanding, you will teach your teen valuable lessons in empathy, resilience, and emotional intelligence.

Communicating with your teen during their hormonal years may not always be easy, but by approaching conversations with empathy, patience, and Superconscious awareness, you can foster a strong, supportive relationship built on trust and understanding. So, roll up your sleeves, buckle up, and get ready to navigate the hormonal highways of adolescence with confidence and grace.

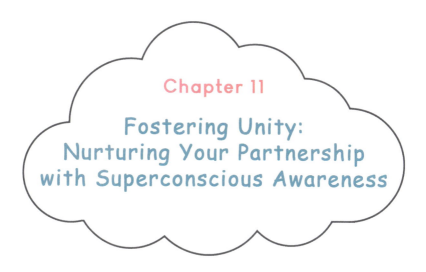

Chapter 11

Fostering Unity:
Nurturing Your Partnership
with Superconscious Awareness

Ah, love! A timeless dance of connection, intimacy, and partnership that enriches our lives and fuels our souls. This chapter will explore the art of nurturing your relationship with your spouse or partner with grace, compassion, and Superconscious Swagger. From effective communication to prioritizing quality time together, get ready to deepen your bond and reignite the spark of love with Superconscious Swagger.

Welcome to a chapter dedicated to nurturing a healthy, vibrant relationship with your partner and embracing your journey of love with Superconscious Swagger. This chapter will explore the keys to cultivating harmony, fostering connections, and infusing your partnership with joy, passion, and purpose.

Your relationship with your partner is the cornerstone of your family's foundation, the bedrock upon which your shared dreams and aspirations are built, but maintaining a thriving partnership requires intention, effort, and a sprinkle of Superconscious Swagger.

With Superconscious Swagger, you can cultivate a relationship grounded in love, trust, and mutual respect. By prioritizing communication, connection, and shared experiences, you can deepen your bond with your partner and create a resilient, fulfilling partnership built to last.

Fostering Unity

So, how can you nurture your relationship with Superconscious Swagger? Here are a few tips to help you get started:

1. **Prioritize Quality Time:** Carve out dedicated time each day to connect with your spouse or partner, whether over a leisurely dinner, a sunset walk, or a cozy movie night at home. Quality time doesn't have to be extravagant—it's about being present, attentive, and fully engaged in each other's company.

2. **Communicate with Compassion**: Effective communication is the cornerstone of a healthy relationship. Practice active listening, empathy, and vulnerability when communicating with your spouse or partner, and strive to express your needs, desires, and feelings openly and honestly.

3. **Show Appreciation**: Express gratitude for your spouse or partner and their role in your life. Whether it's a simple thank

you for washing the dishes or a heartfelt note expressing your love and appreciation, small gestures can go a long way in strengthening your bond.

4. **Keep the Romance Alive:** Don't let the spark fade in your relationship. Keep the romance alive with thoughtful gestures, surprise date nights, and spontaneous acts of affection. Show your spouse or partner they're still the love of your life, and make an effort to keep the passion and excitement alive in your partnership.

5. **Cultivate Shared Goals and Dreams**: Work with your spouse or partner to identify shared goals, dreams, and aspirations for your life together. Whether it's planning a dream vacation, saving for a new home, or pursuing a shared hobby or interest, having common goals can strengthen your bond and deepen your connection.

6. **Seek Support When Needed**: Don't be afraid to seek outside support when needed, whether it's through couples therapy, marriage counseling, or relationship coaching. Asking for help is a sign of strength, not weakness, and seeking support can help you navigate challenges and strengthen your relationship.

Remember that nurturing a healthy relationship with your spouse or partner is a journey, not a destination. By consciously approaching your partnership with intention and love, you can create a relationship filled with joy, passion, and purpose, one that truly stands the test of time.

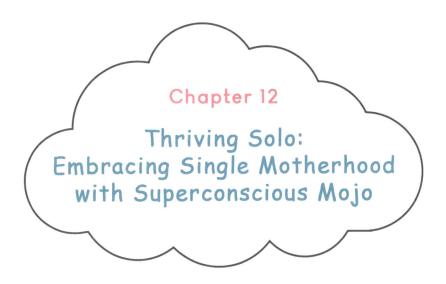

Chapter 12

Thriving Solo: Embracing Single Motherhood with Superconscious Mojo

Welcome to a chapter dedicated to all the remarkable single moms navigating the joys and challenges of parenthood alone. This chapter will explore tips, strategies, and Superconscious techniques for thriving as a single mom. From prioritizing self-care to embracing independence, get ready to embrace your role with confidence, resilience, and Superconscious Swagger.

Welcome to a chapter dedicated to all the incredible single moms navigating the joys and challenges of parenthood alone. In this chapter, we explore the unique journey of single parenthood and share tips and strategies for embracing your role as a single mom while prioritizing your own growth, happiness, and fulfillment, with a touch of Superconscious Swagger.

Embracing Single Motherhood with Superconscious Mojo

As a single mom, you're no stranger to balancing work, parenting, and self-care, but with a little Superconscious Swagger, you'll be able to navigate this journey with confidence, clarity, and purpose. So, how can you consciously thrive as a single mom? Here are a few tips to help you get started:

1. **Prioritize Self-Care**: As a single mom, it's easy to put your needs on the back burner while focusing on caring for your kids, but self-care is essential for your well-being and resilience as a parent. Make time for activities that nourish your mind, body, and spirit, whether it's practicing yoga, going for a nature walk, or enjoying a quiet cup of tea before bed.

2. **Cultivate Supportive Relationships**: Surround yourself with a supportive community of friends, family members, and a couple of fellow single moms who understand and empathize with your journey. Lean on these relationships for emotional support, practical assistance, and encouragement during challenging times.

3. **Set Boundaries**: Boundaries are essential for maintaining your sanity and preserving your energy as a single mom. Be clear about your needs and limits, and don't be afraid to say no to requests or obligations that don't align with your priorities or values. Remember, it's okay to put yourself first sometimes.

4. **Embrace Independence**: Being a single mom doesn't mean you have to do everything alone. Embrace your independence

and resourcefulness, and don't hesitate to ask for help. Whether hiring a babysitter for a much-needed break or delegating household chores to your teens, don't be afraid to lean on others for support.

5. **Get Back Out There**: If you're ready to start meeting new people and exploring the possibility of dating again, don't let fear hold you back. Put yourself out there with confidence and Superconscious Swagger, whether through online dating, social events, or joining a new hobby or interest group. Remember, love and making new connections are possible at any age and stage of life.

6. **Focus on Your Goals**: As a single mom, it's easy to get caught up in the day-to-day challenges of parenting and lose sight of your goals and aspirations. Reflect on your dreams and priorities, and set concrete goals for your personal and professional growth. Whether pursuing further education, advancing in your career, or starting a new business, don't be afraid to dream big and take bold action toward your goals.

Remember, ladies, that being a single mom is both challenging and rewarding. By embracing your role with a little Superconscious mojo, you can navigate the ups and downs of single parenthood with grace, resilience, and a sense of purpose. So, embrace the adventure of single parenthood with open arms, a heart full of love, and a sprinkle of Superconscious Swagger!

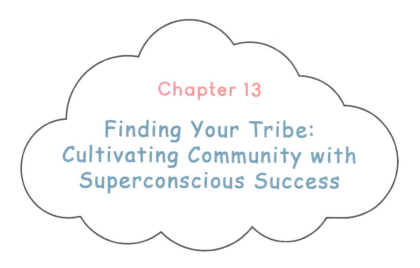

Chapter 13

**Finding Your Tribe:
Cultivating Community with
Superconscious Success**

Welcome to a chapter dedicated to the power of community and connection in your journey toward Superconscious living. This chapter will explore the importance of surrounding yourself with like-minded individuals, who will uplift, support, and inspire you. From fostering deep friendships to finding your tribe, embrace the magic of community with open arms and Superconscious Swagger.

This chapter will explore the importance of building strong connections, the transformative power of friendships and community, and how surrounding yourself with like-minded individuals can elevate your journey to Superconscious living.

We can all agree that life is better when shared with good friends and a supportive community. As a mom, you may often find yourself juggling various responsibilities and navigating the complexities of family life, but amidst the chaos, it's essential to prioritize nurturing relationships with friends and surrounding yourself with like-minded mothers.

Good friends are like sunshine on a cloudy day: they brighten your spirits, lift your mood, and remind you that you're never alone. Whether it's sharing a laugh over coffee, lending a listening ear during challenging times, or celebrating life's victories together, friends enrich our lives in countless ways, but the benefits of friendship extend beyond mere companionship.

Research has shown that strong social connections are linked to better mental and physical health, increased happiness, and longevity. By cultivating meaningful friendships and building a supportive community, you'll enhance your well-being and resilience and create a safety net for navigating life's ups and downs.

Tips for Building Your Tribe:

1. **Seek Out Local Mom Groups**: Look for local mom groups or parenting clubs in your area where you can connect with other mothers facing similar challenges and joys. These groups often host playdates, workshops, and social events that provide opportunities for bonding and support.

2. **Attend Community Events**: Get involved in community events and activities where you're likely to meet other mothers with shared interests. Whether it's a neighborhood picnic, a charity fundraiser, or a fitness class, participating in community

events can help you expand your social circle and find fellow moms to connect with.

3. **Join Online Communities**: Explore online forums, social media groups, and parenting websites where you can connect with other moms virtually. These online communities offer a convenient way to exchange advice, share experiences, and support one another, regardless of geographical location.

4. **Be Open and Authentic**: When meeting new moms, be open and authentic about your experiences, challenges, and aspirations. Vulnerability breeds connection, so don't be afraid to share your journey and listen to others' stories with empathy and understanding.

5. **Fostering Connections**: Invest time and effort in cultivating bonds with other moms by regularly reaching out, checking in, and offering support when needed. Attend meetups, coffee dates, or moms' nights out to stay connected and strengthen your bonds over time.

By following these tips and actively seeking opportunities to connect with other like-minded moms, you can build a supportive community that will uplift and empower your motherhood journey.

So, go ahead—embrace your tribe of friends and community with open arms. Together, you can harness the power of connection to create a life filled with joy, abundance, and positive relationships.

PART 3

Mom's Well-Being Makeover: Aligning Mind, Body, and Purpose

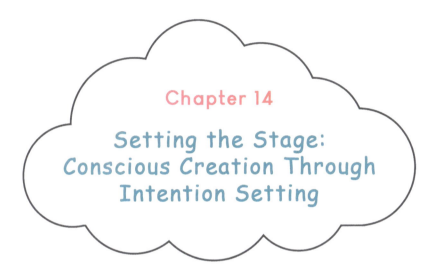

Chapter 14

Setting the Stage: Conscious Creation Through Intention Setting

It's time to channel your inner superhero and set some intentions! We'll dive into the art of goal setting with a twist of Superconscious Swagger. Forget about vague wishes; we're talking about clear, concise intentions that will light the path to your dreams. Prepare to declare to the universe, "I'm coming for you!"

Welcome back to the next chapter in your journey to Superconscious living! In this chapter, we roll up our sleeves, put on our Supermom capes, and dive headfirst into the art of intention setting, but not just any intention setting: intention setting with a twist of Superconscious Swagger.

First, let's address the elephant in the room: intentions versus wishes. How often have you found yourself wishing for something—a better job, a healthier body, more meaningful relationships—only to have your wishes fall flat, like deflated balloons floating away into the abyss? We've all been there, but fear not! With the power of intention setting, you can turn your wishes into reality and transform your dreams into tangible goals.

The Power of Intention

What, exactly, is intention setting, and why is it so powerful? At its core, intention setting is about declaring to the universe what you desire and aligning your thoughts, beliefs, and actions with that desire. It's about planting seeds of possibility in the fertile soil of your mind and nurturing them with love, faith, and perseverance until they blossom into reality.

Think of intention setting as a roadmap for your dreams, a guiding light that illuminates the path forward and keeps you focused, motivated, and inspired. With clear, concise intentions, you can cut through the noise of everyday life and zero in on what truly matters to you, allowing you to make decisions, take action, and overcome obstacles with confidence and clarity.

Superconscious Swagger: The Secret Sauce

Here's the twist: we're not just talking about any old intentions—we're talking about intentions infused with Superconscious Swagger, that inner fire, that unshakable confidence, that unwavering belief in yourself and your ability to create the life of your dreams.

Superconscious Swagger is about stepping into your power as a creator, a co-conspirator with the universe in the grand adventure of life. It's about owning your worth, trusting your intuition, and daring to dream big, audacious, soul-stirring dreams. With Superconscious Swagger, you're not just setting intentions; you're declaring to the universe, "I'm here, I'm ready, and I'm coming for you!"

Crafting Your Superconscious Intentions

Now that we understand the power of intention setting and the magic of Superconscious Swagger, it's time to roll up our sleeves and craft some intentions that will light the path to our dreams. Here are five strategies to get you started:

1. **Get Clear:** Take the time to understand your desire. What are your heart's deepest desires? What would you love to create, experience, or achieve in your life? Write it down, and don't hold back!

2. **Be Specific:** Once you've identified your desires, get specific about what you want. Instead of saying, "I want to be happy," try saying, "I intend to cultivate deep, lasting happiness in my life by prioritizing self-care, nurturing my relationships, and pursuing my passions."

3. **Set a Deadline:** Give your intentions some teeth by setting a deadline for their manifestation. When do you want to achieve your goal? Be realistic, but also stretch yourself to reach beyond your comfort zone.

4. **Visualize Success:** Close your eyes and visualize yourself achieving your intention. What does it look like? How does it feel? Imagine yourself stepping into the reality of your dreams and embodying the person you want to become.

5. **Take Inspired Action:** Take inspired action toward your intention. Break it down into smaller, manageable steps, and take consistent action toward your daily goal. Trust that the universe will support you every step of the way.

Putting It into Practice

Now that you've crafted your Superconscious intentions, it's time to put them into practice. Here are a few tips to help you stay on track:

1. **Stay Focused:** Keep your intentions front and center in your mind and heart. Write them down, post them somewhere you'll see them every day, and repeat them to yourself often.

2. **Stay Flexible:** Life is full of twists and turns, and sometimes, our plans don't unfold exactly as we'd hoped. Stay flexible and open to new opportunities and possibilities that may arise along the way.

3. **Stay Persistent:** Rome wasn't built in a day, and neither are your dreams. Stay persistent and resilient in the face of obstacles and setbacks, and never lose sight of the vision you're working toward.

4. **Stay Grateful:** Finally, stay grateful for the blessings and opportunities that come your way even before your intentions fully manifest. Cultivate an attitude of gratitude and watch as the universe conspires to bring even more abundance into your life.

Congratulations, you've set the stage for Superconscious success! By crafting clear, concise intentions infused with Superconscious Swagger, you've declared to the universe that you're ready to create the life of your dreams. So, go ahead—dream big, aim high, and get ready to conquer the world with your Superconscious intentions!

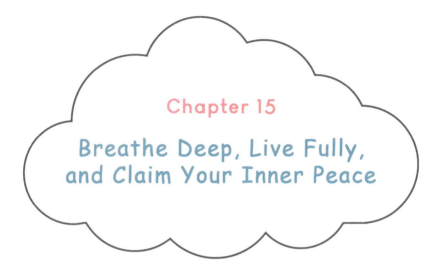

Chapter 15

Breathe Deep, Live Fully, and Claim Your Inner Peace

Who knew something as simple as breathing could be so darn powerful? In this chapter, we explore the transformative magic of deep breathing. Think of it as a mini vacation for your soul, a chance to press pause, recalibrate, and tap into your Superconscious inner peace with each inhale and exhale.

Amidst the hustle and bustle of our daily lives, we'll embark on a journey to discover the profound power of deep breathing, a simple yet potent tool for cultivating inner peace, clarity, and vitality.

The Art of Deep Breathing

Before practicing deep breathing, let's take a moment to understand what it is and why it's so important. Deep breathing, also known as abdominal breathing, is a technique involving breathing deeply into the lower lungs, allowing the diaphragm to expand and contract with each breath fully. If you're anything like how I used to be, I thought a deep breath was when you breathed in and lifted your shoulders up to your ears; this, unfortunately, is known as shallow breathing!

Unlike shallow breathing, which tends to be rapid and confined to the chest, deep breathing engages the diaphragm. It activates the body's relaxation response, triggering a cascade of physiological and psychological benefits. As we breathe deeply, we oxygenate the body, release muscle tension, and calm the mind, promoting a sense of calm, clarity, and well-being.

The Benefits of Deep Breathing

What are the benefits of incorporating deep breathing into our daily lives? The list is long, but here are a few of the many ways deep breathing can enhance our physical, mental, and emotional health:

- **Promotes Relaxation:** Deep breathing activates the body's relaxation response, helping to reduce levels of stress hormones such as cortisol and promote a sense of calm and tranquility.

- **Reduces Anxiety:** Deep breathing has been shown to reduce symptoms of anxiety and panic disorders by calming the nervous system and soothing the mind.

- **Improves Focus and Concentration:** Oxygenating the brain increases blood flow to the prefrontal cortex, which plays a crucial role in executive functioning, such as decision-making and focusing attention. This means deep breathing can improve cognitive function, enhance focus, and sharpen mental clarity.

- **Boosts Energy and Vitality:** Deep breathing increases oxygen delivery to the cells, fueling the body with energy and promoting a sense of alertness and vitality.

- **Supports Emotional Well-being:** Deep breathing helps regulate emotions, reduces feelings of anger, frustration, and irritability, and promotes a greater sense of emotional balance and resilience.

Superconscious Swagger: The Secret Ingredient

Here's the twist: we're not just talking about any old deep breathing—we're talking about deep breathing infused with Superconscious Swagger. How, exactly, does Superconscious Swagger affect deep breathing? It's all about approaching each breath with intention, mindfulness, and a deep sense of reverence for the miraculous gift of life.

Superconscious Swagger is about tapping into the wisdom of your Superconscious mind, the part of your consciousness that transcends the limitations of your ego and connects you to a higher source of wisdom, guidance, and healing. By infusing your deep breathing practice with Superconscious Swagger, you can tap into a deep reservoir of inner peace, clarity, and vitality that empowers you to live fully and vibrantly.

Harnessing the Power of Deep Breathing

Now that we understand the transformative potential of deep breathing and the magic of Superconscious Swagger, let's explore some practical techniques for incorporating deep breathing into your daily routine. Here are a few simple yet potent techniques to get you started:

1. **Abdominal Breathing:** Begin by finding a comfortable seated or lying position. Place one hand on your chest and the other on your abdomen. Take a slow, deep breath through your nose, allowing your abdomen to fully expand as you inhale. Then, exhale slowly through your mouth, allowing your abdomen to contract. Continue to breathe deeply and rhythmically, noticing the sensation of your breath moving in and out of your body.

2. **4-7-8 Breath:** This technique, popularized by Dr. Andrew Weil, is a simple yet powerful way to promote relaxation and reduce stress. Begin by exhaling through your mouth loudly enough to hear it. Then, close your mouth and inhale quietly through your nose for a count of four. Hold your breath for a count of seven. Finally, exhale slowly and audibly through your mouth for a count of eight, making a whooshing sound. Repeat this cycle for four rounds until you feel calm and relaxed.

3. **Alternate Nostril Breathing:** This ancient yogic technique balances the left and right hemispheres of the brain, promotes mental clarity, and soothes the nervous system. Begin by sitting comfortably with your spine straight, and your shoulders relaxed. Place your left hand on your left knee with your palm facing up. Bring your right hand up to your nose and place your thumb on your right nostril and your ring finger or pinky finger on your left nostril. Close your right nostril with your thumb and inhale deeply through your left nostril. Then, close your left nostril with your ring or pinky finger and exhale through your right nostril. Inhale through your right nostril, then close it with your thumb and exhale through your left nostril. Continue this pattern for several rounds, alternating nostrils with each breath.

4. **Breath Counting:** This practice involves counting your breaths to focus your attention and quiet the mind. Begin by finding a comfortable seated position and closing your eyes. Take a deep breath in through your nose, counting "one" silently in your mind. Then, exhale slowly through your nose, counting "two." Continue to inhale and exhale, counting each breath to ten, then start again at one. If you lose count or become distracted, simply return to one and begin again. This practice can help cultivate mindfulness, presence, and concentration while promoting relaxation and stress relief.

Putting It into Practice

Now that you have a toolbox full of Superconscious deep breathing techniques, it's time to put them into practice. Here's a step-by-step guide to help you harness the power of deep breathing and live fully:

1. **Set Aside Time:** Find a quiet, comfortable space to practice deep breathing without distractions. Set aside dedicated time each day to engage in your deep breathing practice, whether it's first thing in the morning, during your lunch break, or before bed.

2. **Get Comfortable:** Find a comfortable seated or lying position that allows you to relax and breathe deeply. You may sit cross-legged on the floor, sit in a chair with your feet flat on the ground, or lie down on your back with your arms resting by your sides.

3. **Focus Your Attention:** Close your eyes and bring your attention to your breath. Notice the sensation of the breath moving in and out of your body, the rise and fall of your chest or abdomen, the feeling of air passing through your nostrils, and the sound of your breath as it enters and exits your body.

4. **Choose Your Technique:** Choose a deep breathing technique from the ones we've explored—or any other technique that resonates with you—and practice it. Experiment with different techniques to see which are most effective and enjoyable.

5. **Practice Mindfulness:** As you practice deep breathing, practice mindfulness by staying present and attentive to each breath. Notice any thoughts or feelings that arise without judgment or attachment, and gently guide your attention back to the breath whenever you become distracted.

6. **Stay Consistent:** Consistency is key when deep breathing. Commit to practicing your chosen technique regularly, even if you don't feel stressed, to build resilience and cultivate a sense of inner peace and well-being.

7. **Integrate into Daily Life:** Finally, integrate deep breathing into your daily life by incorporating it into moments of stress, tension, or feeling overwhelmed. Whenever you feel yourself becoming stressed or anxious, take a few moments to pause, breathe deeply, and reconnect with your breath. Remember, the power to calm your mind, soothe your nerves, and live fully is always within you—all you must do is breathe.

Congratulations, you've unlocked the power of deep breathing! By harnessing the transformative magic of deep breathing and infusing it with Superconscious Swagger, you're tapping into a deep well of inner peace, clarity, and vitality that will empower you to live fully and vibrantly. So, go ahead—breathe deeply, live fully, and embrace the boundless possibilities that await you with each inhale and exhale!

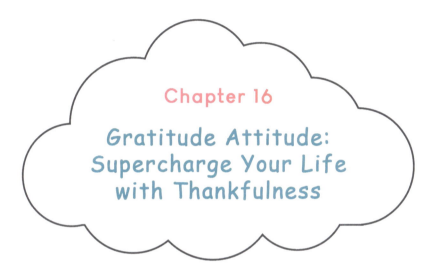

Chapter 16

Gratitude Attitude:
Supercharge Your Life
with Thankfulness

Gratitude: it's like glitter for the soul! In this chapter, we'll sprinkle a generous dose of thankfulness into your life and watch the magic unfold. From gratitude journals to daily appreciation rituals, we'll show you how to cultivate a gratitude attitude that attracts blessings like bees to honey.

Welcome to gratitude attitude—where we embark on a journey to supercharge your life with the transformative power of thankfulness. In a world filled with hustle and bustle, stress, and striving, cultivating gratitude offers a beacon of light—a reminder to pause, reflect, and appreciate the abundant blessings surrounding us each day.

The Power of Gratitude

Before we dive into the practical strategies for cultivating a gratitude attitude, let's take a moment to explore why gratitude is such a powerful force for good in our lives. Gratitude, my friends, is more than just a fleeting feeling of thankfulness; it's a way of seeing the world, a lens through which we view life's challenges and blessings with clarity, humility, and appreciation.

Countless studies have shown that practicing gratitude can profoundly affect physical, mental, and emotional well-being. From reducing stress and anxiety levels to promoting feelings of happiness and contentment, the benefits of gratitude are far-reaching and scientifically validated.

Cultivating a Gratitude Attitude

So, how can we cultivate a gratitude attitude and harness the transformative power of thankfulness in our daily lives? Fortunately, there are countless ways to cultivate gratitude—all it takes is a willingness to open your heart and mind to the abundance of blessings surrounding you each day. Here are a few simple yet potent strategies to get you started:

1. **Gratitude Journaling:** Keep a gratitude journal, a space dedicated to recording three to five things you're grateful for daily. Whether it's a beautiful sunrise, a kind gesture from a stranger, or a moment of laughter with loved ones, take a few minutes each day to reflect on the blessings in your life and write them down. Over time, you'll notice patterns of

abundance and beauty emerging in your life, reinforcing your gratitude attitude and attracting even more blessings.

2. **Daily Appreciation Rituals:** Incorporate daily appreciation rituals into your routine to cultivate a sense of thankfulness and mindfulness throughout the day. Whether starting your morning with gratitude, expressing appreciation for your meals, or reflecting on your day before bed, find moments throughout the day to pause, breathe, and savor the blessings surrounding you.

3. **Gratitude Walks:** Take gratitude walks in nature to connect with the beauty and abundance of the natural world and cultivate feelings of awe, wonder, and thankfulness. Whether it's a stroll through a local park, a hike in the mountains, or a leisurely walk along the beach, immerse yourself in the sights, sounds, and sensations of nature and express gratitude for the abundance of life surrounding you.

4. **Gratitude Letters:** Write gratitude letters to express appreciation for the people in your life who have had a positive impact on you. Whether it's a friend, family member, mentor, or colleague, take the time to write a heartfelt letter expressing gratitude for their kindness, support, and friendship. Not only will this practice deepen your connections with others, but it will also fill your heart with warmth and gratitude.

5. **Gratitude Meditation:** Practice gratitude meditation to cultivate feelings of thankfulness and appreciation in your heart and mind. Find a comfortable space to sit or lie down without distractions and close your eyes. Take a few deep breaths, relax, and let go of any tension or stress. Then, recall three to five things you're grateful for, allowing yourself to savor the feelings of appreciation and thankfulness with each breath.

Putting It into Practice

Now that you have a toolbox full of gratitude practices, it's time to experience the magic of gratitude firsthand. Here's a step-by-step guide to help you cultivate a gratitude attitude and supercharge your life with thankfulness:

1. **Start Small:** Include one or two gratitude practices in your daily routine, such as journaling or meditation. Start small and gradually build momentum over time, allowing yourself to cultivate a habit of thankfulness and appreciation.

2. **Stay Consistent:** Consistency is key to cultivating gratitude. Commit to practicing your chosen gratitude techniques regularly, even when you're not feeling particularly grateful, to build resilience and cultivate a sense of thankfulness and appreciation.

3. **Notice the Little Things:** Take time to notice the little things in life that bring you joy and gratitude: the warmth of the sun on your skin, the sound of birds singing in the morning, or the taste of your favorite meal. Cultivate a sense of wonder and awe for the simple pleasures surrounding you each day, and express gratitude for the abundance of beauty and blessings in your life.

4. **Shift Your Perspective:** Use gratitude as a lens through which to view life's challenges and blessings with clarity, humility, and appreciation. Instead of focusing on what's lacking or missing in your life, shift your perspective to focus on the abundance and blessings surrounding you, even amidst adversity.

5. **Share Your Gratitude:** Finally, share your gratitude with others by expressing appreciation for the people, experiences, and blessings in your life. Whether it's a heartfelt thank you to a loved one or a simple act of kindness,

spread gratitude wherever you go and watch as the magic of thankfulness unfolds in your life and the lives of those around you.

The Ripple Effect of Gratitude

As you cultivate a gratitude attitude and supercharge your life with thankfulness, you'll notice a ripple effect of positivity and abundance spreading throughout every aspect of your life. You'll attract more blessings, opportunities, and synchronicities into your life and experience greater levels of happiness, fulfillment, and well-being.

So, go ahead—embrace the magic of gratitude, cultivate a gratitude attitude, and watch as your life transforms before your very eyes. With each moment of thankfulness, you'll plant seeds of abundance and joy that will bloom and flourish in the garden of your heart, filling your life with beauty, blessings, and boundless possibilities.

Congratulations, you've unlocked the transformative power of gratitude! By cultivating a gratitude attitude and supercharging your life with thankfulness, you're embracing a life of abundance, joy, and infinite possibility. Feel free to sprinkle gratitude like glitter in your life and watch the magic unfold in every moment of every day.

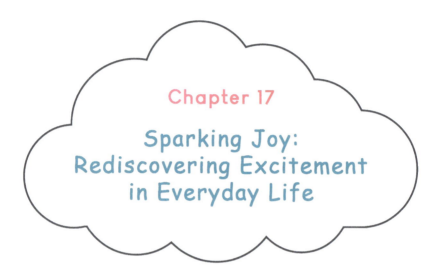

Chapter 17

**Sparking Joy:
Rediscovering Excitement
in Everyday Life**

Are you tired of feeling stuck in the same old routine? Do you long for a sense of excitement and adventure in your life? In this chapter, we explore strategies for reigniting the spark of joy and passion in your days, from planning family trips to embracing your creative side and learning something new. Get ready to infuse your life with excitement and rediscover the thrill of living each day to the fullest!

Welcome to a chapter dedicated to reigniting the spark of excitement and passion in your life. Getting caught up in the whirlwind of daily routines and responsibilities is too easy, leaving you feeling stuck and uninspired, but within you is the power to infuse your days with joy, creativity, and adventure.

Adding Excitement to Your Life

There are so many ways to infuse your life with excitement and joy; here are a few practices to get you started:

1. **Planning family trips and adventures**: Whether it's a weekend getaway to a nearby city, a camping trip in the great outdoors, a fun-filled day at an amusement park, or catching a sunset at the beach, taking the time to explore new places and create lasting memories with your loved ones can breathe new life into your days.

2. **Embracing Your Creative Side**: Do you enjoy singing, dancing, playing an instrument, or getting crafty at paint night? Finding activities that ignite your passion and bring you joy can help break up the monotony of daily life and infuse your days with excitement and inspiration.

3. **Acquiring New Skills**: Learning something new is a powerful way to add excitement and meaning to your life. Try picking up a new hobby, learning another language, or enrolling in a class that interests you, challenging yourself to step outside of your comfort zone and expand your horizons can reignite your sense of curiosity and wonder.

4. **Incorporating Small Joys**: Embracing simple pleasures can bring excitement back into your life. Taking time to savor the little things, like testing new recipes at family dinners, going for a walk with your dog, or spending time in nature, can help you reconnect with the beauty and magic of the world around you.

Know that you have the power to add excitement and joy back into your life, no matter how stuck or uninspired you may feel. By welcoming new experiences, nurturing your creativity, and savoring the simple pleasures of everyday life, you can reignite the spark of passion and purpose within you. So, go ahead—embrace the excitement of living with open arms, and let your light shine brightly in the world!

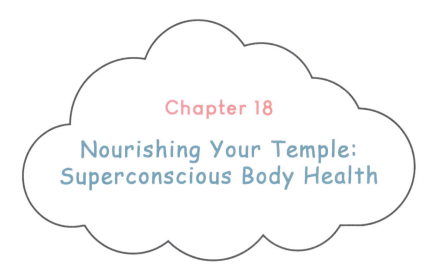

Chapter 18

Nourishing Your Temple: Superconscious Body Health

Ah, the sweet symphony of a well-nourished body! In this chapter, we whip up a recipe for radiant health infused with Superconscious Swagger. From leafy greens to soul-nourishing treats, we explore how to fuel your body to honor your inner goddess (or superhero—your choice!).

It's time to nourish your temple. Here, we embark on a journey of culinary delights, exploring the art of nourishing your body with intention, mindfulness, and a healthy dose of Superconscious Swagger.

The Importance of Nourishment

Before we dive into the specifics of nourishing your body, let's take a moment to appreciate food's profound impact on our overall health and well-being. Our bodies are temples—sacred vessels that house our minds, spirits, and souls—and it's our responsibility to care for them with love, respect, and gratitude.

Nourishment goes beyond mere sustenance. It's about feeding our bodies the nutrients they need to thrive, flourish, and radiate with vitality. When we nourish our bodies with wholesome, nutrient-dense foods, we're not just fueling our physical bodies; we're nourishing our minds, uplifting our spirits, and honoring the divine within us.

Superconscious Swagger: The Secret Ingredient

Here's the twist, ladies: we're not just talking about any old nourishment but about nourishment infused with Superconscious Swagger. What exactly does that mean regarding nourishing your body? It's all about approaching food with intention, mindfulness, and a deep reverence for the miraculous vessel that is your body.

Superconscious Swagger is about listening to your body's innate wisdom and honoring its unique needs and preferences, choosing foods that nourish not just your physical body but also your mind, spirit, and soul. It's about cultivating a healthy relationship with food based on joy, pleasure, and self-care rather than guilt, restriction, or deprivation.

Fueling Your Body with Superconscious Swagger

Now that we understand the importance of nourishing our bodies with the power of Superconscious Swagger, let's explore some practical strategies for fueling your body in a way that honors your inner goddess (or superhero—your choice!). Here are a few tips to get you started:

1. **Eat Whole, Nutrient-Dense Foods:** Focus on incorporating whole, nutrient-dense foods into your diet, such as fruit, vegetables, whole grains, lean proteins, and healthy fats. These foods are packed with essential vitamins, minerals, and antioxidants that nourish your body from the inside out.

2. **Listen to Your Body:** Pay attention to how different foods make you feel and honor your body's unique signals and cravings. If a particular food energizes, satisfies, and nourishes, keep it in your rotation. If it leaves you feeling sluggish, bloated, or uncomfortable, consider whether it's worth including in your diet.

3. **Practice Mindful Eating:** Slow down and savor each bite of food, paying attention to the flavors, textures, and sensations as you eat. Mindful eating helps you enjoy your food more fully and allows you to tune into your body's hunger and fullness cues, preventing overeating and promoting greater satisfaction.

4. **Stay Hydrated:** Drink plenty of water throughout the day to stay hydrated and support your body's natural detoxification processes. Aim for at least eight glasses of water daily, and consider incorporating hydrating foods such as fruit, vegetables, and herbal teas into your diet.

5. **Practice Moderation:** While nourishing your body with wholesome, nutrient-dense food is important, it's also important to indulge in moderation. Allow yourself to occasionally enjoy your favorite treats and indulgences without

guilt or shame. Remember, balance is the key to maintaining a healthy relationship with food.

Putting It into Practice

Now that you have a solid understanding of Superconscious Swagger and some practical tips for nourishing your body, it's time to put them into practice. Here's a step-by-step guide to help you get started:

1. **Stock Your Pantry:** Start by stocking your pantry and refrigerator with wholesome, nutrient-dense foods that nourish your body and satisfy your taste buds. Fill your kitchen with a rainbow of fruit, vegetables, whole grains, lean proteins, and healthy fats.

2. **Plan Your Meals:** Take some time each week to plan your meals and snacks, considering your schedule, preferences, and dietary needs. Batch cook and meal prep whenever possible to save time and ensure healthy options are always available when hunger strikes.

3. **Listen to Your Body:** Tune into your body's hunger and fullness cues and honor its unique needs and preferences. Eat when you're hungry, stop when you're full, and enjoy your food without judgment or restriction.

4. **Practice Mindful Eating:** Slow down and savor each bite of food, paying attention to the flavors, textures, and sensations as you eat. Put away distractions such as phones, computers, and TVs, and focus fully on eating.

5. **Stay Hydrated:** Drink plenty of water throughout the day to stay hydrated and support your body's natural detoxification processes. Carry a reusable water bottle wherever you go, and sip on water regularly throughout the day.

6. **Practice Gratitude:** Practice gratitude for the nourishment you receive, whether from a home-cooked meal, a nutritious snack, or a refreshing glass of water. Cultivate an attitude of gratitude for the abundance of nourishing food available to you, and savor each bite with joy and appreciation.

Congratulations, you've unlocked the secret to radiant health and vitality! By nourishing your body with intention, mindfulness, and a healthy dose of Superconscious Swagger, you're honoring the sacred vessel that is your body and fueling yourself for a life filled with energy, vitality, and joy. So, go ahead, ladies—whip up a delicious meal, savor each bite, and embrace the nourishing power of Superconscious Swagger!

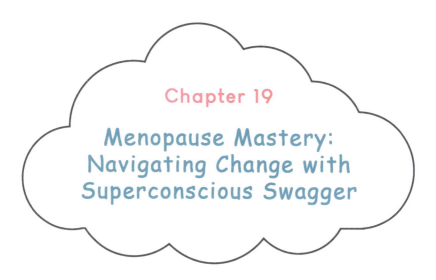

Chapter 19

Menopause Mastery: Navigating Change with Superconscious Swagger

Ah, menopause — the inevitable journey of change that every woman faces as she transitions through midlife. Fear not, dear moms, in this chapter, we equip you with the tools, techniques, and strategies needed to navigate this transformative time with grace, confidence, and a sense of empowerment. Get ready to embrace the wisdom of your body and step into this new chapter of life with poise and Superconscious Swagger.

Welcome to a chapter dedicated to navigating the tumultuous waters of menopause with grace, resilience, and a little Superconscious Swagger, where we explore the transformative journey of menopause and share practical tips for embracing change and thriving during this transition.

Menopause is a natural and inevitable stage of life for women, yet it's often accompanied by physical and emotional changes that can leave you feeling overwhelmed, confused, and out of sorts. However, menopause is also an opportunity for growth, empowerment, and self-discovery.

With a sprinkle of Superconscious Swagger, you can navigate the menopause maze confidently and gracefully. By embracing change as a natural part of life and adopting a positive mindset, you can transform this transition into a time of renewal, reinvention, and rediscovery.

Menopause Mastery

How can you harness the power of Superconscious Swagger to navigate menopause with ease and grace? Here are six tips to get you started:

1. **Embrace Self-Care**: Menopause is a time to prioritize self-care and nurture your body, mind, and spirit. Make time for activities that bring you joy and relaxation, whether practicing yoga, meditating, or indulging in a luxurious bubble bath.

2. **Seek Support:** Don't go through menopause alone. Reach out to friends, family, and healthcare professionals for support and guidance. Joining an online community can also provide valuable insights and camaraderie during this change.

3. **Stay Active**: Regular exercise can help alleviate common menopausal symptoms such as hot flashes, mood swings, and insomnia. Aim for at least 30 minutes of moderate-intensity

exercise, whether walking, swimming, or dancing, on most days of the week.

4. **Prioritize Nutrition**: A healthy diet can help ease menopausal symptoms and support overall well-being. Focus on eating a balanced diet rich in fruit, vegetables, whole grains, and lean proteins, and limit your intake of caffeine, alcohol, and processed foods.

5. **Practice Mindfulness**: Mindfulness techniques, such as deep breathing, meditation, and visualization, can help reduce stress, anxiety, and other menopausal symptoms. Incorporate these practices into your daily routine to cultivate inner peace and resilience.

6. **Embrace Change**: Instead of resisting or fearing change, embrace it as an opportunity for growth and transformation. Embrace your evolving body and embrace the wisdom that comes with age, knowing that you are strong, adaptable, and capable of navigating any challenge that comes your way.

By embracing change with Superconscious Swagger, you can navigate the menopause maze with confidence, grace, and resilience. Remember that you're not alone on this journey. With the support of your tribe and the power of your inner wisdom, you can embrace menopause as a time of empowerment, renewal, and transformation.

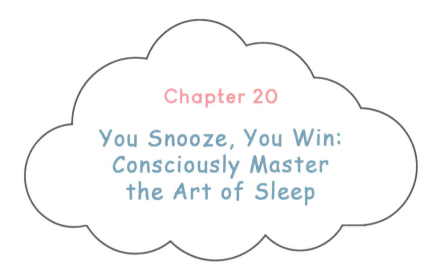

Chapter 20

**You Snooze, You Win:
Consciously Master
the Art of Sleep**

Whoever said sleep is for the weak clearly never experienced the power of a good night's rest! In this chapter, we explore the art of sleep hygiene and teach you how to snooze your way to success with Superconscious Swagger. So, fluff those pillows, dim the lights, and prepare for a night of blissful slumber.

For now, we will put aside the old saying of, "You snooze, you lose," and replace it with you snooze, you win. This is an exploration of the transformative power of sleep and the art of mastering Superconscious sleep hygiene. In a world that often glorifies busyness and productivity, prioritizing sleep can feel like a radical act of self-care, a declaration that your well-being matters just as much as your to-do list. So, snuggle under the covers, close your eyes, and embark on a journey of rest, rejuvenation, and sweet dreams.

The Importance of Sleep

Before we dive into the practical strategies for mastering Superconscious sleep hygiene, let's take a moment to explore why sleep is such a crucial component of well-being and success. Sleep, my friends, is more than a period of rest and relaxation—it's a fundamental biological need that plays a vital role in nearly every aspect of our physical, mental, and emotional health.

During sleep, our bodies repair and regenerate cells, consolidate memories, and process emotions, allowing us to wake up refreshed, energized, and ready to tackle the day ahead. Adequate sleep is also essential for cognitive function, mood regulation, immune function, and overall longevity, making it one of the most important factors in maintaining optimal health and well-being.

The Art of Sleep Hygiene

How can we cultivate Superconscious sleep hygiene, a set of practices and habits that promote restful, rejuvenating sleep and set the stage for success in every area of our lives? Fortunately, there are countless ways to improve your sleep hygiene; all it takes is a willingness to prioritize your well-being and make sleep a non-negotiable part of your daily routine. Here are a few simple yet powerful strategies to get you started:

1. **Establish a Consistent Sleep Schedule:** Go to bed and wake up at the same time every day to regulate your body's internal clock and improve the quality of your sleep. Aim for at least seven hours of sleep each night, and avoid staying up late or sleeping in excessively, as this can disrupt your natural sleep-wake cycle.

2. **Create a Relaxing Bedtime Routine:** Develop a calming bedtime routine to signal to your body that it's time to wind down and prepare for sleep. Engage in relaxing activities such as reading, taking a warm bath or shower, or listening to soothing music to help you relax and unwind before bed.

3. **Optimize Your Sleep Environment:** Create a sleep-friendly environment conducive to restful, rejuvenating sleep. Keep your bedroom cool, dark, and quiet, and minimize noise, light, and distractions.

4. **Limit Exposure to Screens:** Reduce your exposure to screens—such as smartphones, tablets, computers, and televisions—in the hour leading up to bedtime, as the blue light emitted by these devices can interfere with your body's production of melatonin, a hormone that regulates sleep-wake cycles. Instead, engage in relaxing activities promoting sleep, such as reading, journaling, or meditating.

5. **Mind Your Meals and Beverages:** Be mindful of your eating and drinking habits, especially in the hours leading up to bedtime, as it can disrupt your sleep patterns and interfere with your ability to fall asleep and stay asleep.

Putting It into Practice

Now that you understand the importance of sleep and have some strategies for mastering Superconscious sleep hygiene, it's time to put it into practice. Here's a step-by-step guide to help you cultivate a sleep routine that will promote restful, rejuvenating sleep and set the stage for success:

1. **Set a Sleep Schedule:** Establish a consistent sleep schedule by going to bed and waking up at the same time every day, even on weekends (as often as possible!). Aim for at least seven hours of sleep each night and prioritize your bedtime like any other important appointment or commitment.

2. **Create a Bedtime Routine:** Develop a calming bedtime routine that helps you relax and unwind before bed. This could include taking a warm bath or shower, practicing a relaxation technique like deep breathing, or reading a book in bed. Whatever you choose, make sure it's something that helps you transition from the busyness of the day to a state of relaxation and rest.

3. **Optimize Your Sleep Environment:** Make your bedroom a sanctuary for sleep by creating a comfortable and inviting sleep environment. Keep your bedroom cool, dark, and quiet, and invest in high-quality bedding, a supportive mattress, and comfortable pillows. Minimize noise and distractions, and consider using blackout curtains, white noise machines, or earplugs if necessary.

4. **Limit Screen Time:** Reduce your exposure to screens—such as smartphones, tablets, computers, and televisions—in the hour leading up to bedtime. Instead, engage in relaxing activities promoting sleep, such as reading, journaling, or calming music. If you must use screens before bed, consider using blue light-blocking glasses or apps that reduce the blue light emitted by electronic devices.

5. **Mind Your Diet:** Be mindful of your eating and drinking habits, especially in the hours leading up to bedtime. Avoid heavy, spicy, or rich foods that can cause discomfort or indigestion, and limit your intake of caffeine, alcohol, and sugary beverages, as these can disrupt your sleep patterns and interfere with your ability to fall asleep and stay asleep.

The Power of Superconscious Sleep

As you master the art of Superconscious sleep hygiene and prioritize restful, rejuvenating sleep, you'll discover a newfound sense of vitality, clarity, and well-being that will transform every aspect of your life. You'll wake up feeling refreshed, energized, and ready to tackle the day ahead with a renewed sense of purpose and passion for life.

So, fluff those pillows, dim the lights, and embrace the power of Superconscious sleep. With each night of restful slumber, you're nourishing your mind, body, and spirit with love, care, and compassion and laying the foundation for a life filled with health, happiness, and success.

Congratulations, you've unlocked the secrets of Superconscious sleep hygiene! By prioritizing restful, rejuvenating sleep, you're embracing a life of vitality, clarity, and well-being that honors your body's natural rhythms and supports your overall health and happiness. So go ahead—snooze your way to success, and watch as your life unfolds in beautiful, unexpected ways.

PART 4

Elevate Your Swagger: Superconscious Science & Manifestation

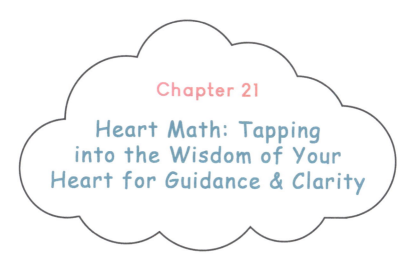

Chapter 21

Heart Math: Tapping into the Wisdom of Your Heart for Guidance & Clarity

Your heart knows best, my friends! Join us as we journey into Heart Math, where science meets soul in a dance of Superconscious wisdom. Get ready to listen to the whispers of your heart and unlock a world of infinite possibility.

Next up is Heart Math—a journey into the depths of your heart's wisdom and the transformative power of living in alignment with your truest desires. Here, amidst the rhythm of our beating hearts, we explore Heart Math's science, philosophy, and practical applications, a revolutionary approach to personal growth, healing, and transformation.

The Heart's Wisdom

Before diving into the world of Heart Math, let's take a moment to appreciate the profound wisdom in our hearts. Far more than a mere pump circulating blood through our bodies, the heart is a powerful organ of perception, intuition, and emotion, a gateway to our deepest truths, desires, and aspirations.

Throughout history, poets, philosophers, and mystics have extolled the wisdom of the heart, recognizing it as the seat of the soul and the source of our greatest insights and inspirations. From Shakespeare's "My heart is ever at your service" to Rumi's "The heart knows a hundred thousand ways to speak," the wisdom of the heart has been celebrated and revered as a guiding light on life's journey.

The Science of Heart Math

As it turns out, science confirms what poets and mystics have known for centuries. The heart is far more than a mere pump; it's a sophisticated organ of perception and intelligence that plays a central role in our physical, mental, and emotional well-being.

In recent decades, scientists at the Institute of Heart Math and other research institutions have conducted groundbreaking research into the science of heart coherence, a state of optimal functioning in which the heart, brain, and nervous system are in harmonious alignment. Through techniques such as heart rate variability (HRV) biofeedback, researchers have demonstrated that cultivating heart coherence can profoundly affect our health, happiness, and overall quality of life.

Heart Math Techniques

So, how can we tap into the wisdom of our hearts and cultivate heart coherence in our daily lives? Enter Heart Math, a revolutionary approach to personal growth and transformation that combines cutting-edge science with ancient wisdom to help us unlock the full potential of our hearts.

At its core, Heart Math is about learning to listen to the whispers of our hearts and aligning our thoughts, feelings, and actions with our deepest truths and desires. Through heart-focused breathing, HRV biofeedback, and heart-centered meditation, we can train ourselves to access the wisdom of our hearts and live in alignment with our truest selves.

Practical Applications

Now that we understand the science and philosophy behind Heart Math, let's explore some practical applications for incorporating these techniques into our daily lives. Here are a few simple yet powerful ways to tap into the wisdom of your heart and live a life of Superconscious awareness:

1. **Heart-Focused Breathing:** Begin by finding a quiet, comfortable space to sit or lie comfortably. Close your eyes and bring your attention to your heart center—the area in the middle of your chest. Take a few deep breaths into your heart center, imagining each breath flowing in and out of your heart like a gentle wave. As you breathe, cultivate feelings of love, gratitude, and compassion in your heart, allowing them to expand with each inhale and exhale.

2. **Heart Rate Variability (HRV) Biofeedback:** HRV biofeedback is a technique involving the use of a biofeedback device to monitor your heart rate variability—variations in the time intervals between heartbeats—and train yourself to increase heart coherence. Start by purchasing an HRV

biofeedback device or using a smartphone app that offers HRV biofeedback. Practice using the device regularly, focusing on slow, rhythmic breathing while cultivating feelings of love, appreciation, and gratitude in your heart. Over time, you'll learn to increase your heart coherence and experience the benefits of improved physical, mental, and emotional well-being.

3. **Heart-Centered Meditation:** Heart-centered meditation is a practice involving bringing your attention to your heart center and cultivating feelings of love, compassion, and appreciation. Begin by finding a comfortable seated position and closing your eyes. Place one hand on your heart and take a few deep breaths into your heart center, allowing yourself to connect with the rhythm of your breath and the beating of your heart. As you breathe deeply, cultivate feelings of love, gratitude, and compassion in your heart, allowing them to radiate outward and fill your entire being with warmth and light.

4. **Heart-Centered Living:** Finally, embrace heart-centered living as a way of life, aligning your thoughts, feelings, and actions with the wisdom of your heart. Listen to the whispers of your heart and follow its guidance, trusting that it knows what is best for you. Cultivate practices of self-love, self-care, and self-compassion, nurturing yourself with the same kindness and compassion you would offer a dear friend. Remember that the wisdom of your heart is always within you, guiding you on your Superconscious journey.

Putting It into Practice

Now that you have a toolbox full of Heart Math techniques, it's time to put them into practice. Here's a step-by-step guide to help you tap into the wisdom of your heart with Superconscious awareness:

1. **Set Aside Time:** Set aside dedicated time each day to engage in your Heart Math practice, whether it's the first thing in the morning, during your lunch break, or before bed. Find a quiet, comfortable space to sit or lie down without distractions, and fully immerse yourself in the practice.

2. **Connect with Your Heart:** Begin each practice by connecting with your heart center, the area in the middle of your chest where your heart resides. Close your eyes and place one hand on your heart, allowing yourself to feel its rhythm and presence. Take a few deep breaths into your heart center, allowing yourself to connect with the wisdom and intelligence of your heart.

3. **Cultivate Feelings of Love and Gratitude:** As you breathe deeply, cultivate love, gratitude, and compassion. Reflect on the people, experiences, and blessings that fill you with love and appreciation, allowing these feelings to expand and radiate outward from your heart.

4. **Practice Heart Math Techniques:** Choose one or more of the Heart Math techniques we've explored—or any other techniques that resonate with you—and practice them regularly. Experiment with different techniques to see which ones feel most effective and enjoyable for you, and don't be afraid to customize your practice to suit your unique needs and preferences.

5. **Integrate into Daily Life:** Finally, integrate Heart Math into your daily life in moments when feeling stressed, tense, or overwhelmed. Whenever you feel yourself becoming stressed or anxious, take a few moments to pause, connect with your heart, and engage in your chosen Heart Math practice. Trust that the wisdom of your heart will guide you on your Superconscious journey, illuminating the path ahead with love, clarity, and grace.

Congratulations, you've unlocked the wisdom of your heart! By tapping into the transformative power of Heart Math and living in alignment with your deepest truths and desires, you're embracing a life of Superconscious living filled with love, joy, and infinite possibility. So, go ahead—listen to the whispers of your heart, follow its guidance, and let your heart lead you on a journey of love, growth, and self-discovery.

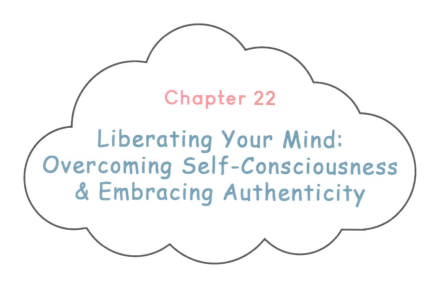

Chapter 22

Liberating Your Mind: Overcoming Self-Consciousness & Embracing Authenticity

Do you ever find yourself comparing your life to the carefully curated images of perfection on social media? In this chapter, we explore the traps of self-consciousness and unveil strategies to break free from its grip. Get ready to embrace your authentic self and live life on your own terms with confidence and authenticity!

Welcome to a chapter dedicated to breaking free from the chains of self-consciousness and embracing the beautiful, imperfect, and authentic essence of who you are. As a busy mom caught in the whirlwind of daily routines, it's all too easy to fall into the trap of comparing yourself to others, especially in the age of social media, but fear not, for the power to reclaim your sense of worth, confidence, and self-love is within you.

Let's explore the self-conscious mind's insidious role in fueling negative thoughts and comparisons. Your self-conscious mind is like a relentless critic, constantly whispering doubts and insecurities into your ear as you scroll through social media feeds filled with curated snapshots of seemingly perfect lives. From the mom who effortlessly juggles work, family, and fitness to the family enjoying an envy-inducing tropical vacation, it's easy to feel inadequate in comparison.

But here's the truth: those picture-perfect moments you see on social media are just a small moment in time. They don't tell the whole story of the struggles, challenges, and imperfections that lie beneath the surface of every family. Yet your self-conscious mind latches onto these images, using them as ammunition to fuel feelings of inadequacy and unworthiness.

So, how do you break free from the grip of self-consciousness and reclaim your sense of authenticity and self-worth? It begins with shifting your mindset and practicing radical self-acceptance. Instead of comparing yourself to others and striving for unattainable standards of perfection, focus on embracing your unique strengths, quirks, and imperfections.

Putting It into Practice

1. **Embrace Self-Love and Self-Compassion**: Treat yourself with the same kindness, understanding, and empathy you would extend to a dear friend. Challenge negative self-talk and replace it with affirmations of love, worthiness, and acceptance.

Remember that you are worthy of love and belonging simply because you exist, not because of how you measure up to others.

2. **Engage in Mindfulness through Meditation**: By cultivating present-moment awareness and observing your thoughts and emotions without judgment, you can detach yourself from the incessant chatter of your self-conscious mind. Practice mindfulness regularly to quiet the noise and cultivate inner peace, clarity, and acceptance.

As you embark on this journey of self-discovery and liberation, remember that progress, not perfection, is the goal. Be patient and compassionate with yourself as you navigate the ups and downs of overcoming self-consciousness. Celebrate your victories, no matter how small, and honor the courage it takes to embrace your authenticity and shine your light brightly in the world.

In conclusion, amazing ladies, know that you are enough, exactly as you are. You are worthy of love, happiness, and fulfillment, and you don't need to compare yourself to anyone else to validate your worth. Embrace your imperfections, celebrate your uniqueness, and remember that true beauty lies in authenticity. So, go ahead— liberate your mind from the shackles of self-consciousness, and step into the fullness of who you are with courage, confidence, and Superconscious Swagger!

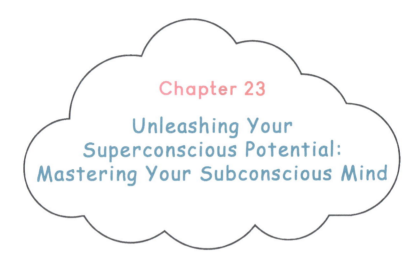

Chapter 23

Unleashing Your Superconscious Potential: Mastering Your Subconscious Mind

Do you ever feel like there's an invisible force holding you back from reaching your full potential? In this chapter, we dive deep into the mysteries of the subconscious mind and uncover how it influences your thoughts, behaviors, and beliefs. Get ready to unlock the power of your subconscious mind and unleash your Superconscious potential like never before!

Welcome to a chapter dedicated to unlocking the power of your subconscious mind and unleashing your Superconscious potential. If you're stuck in the daily grind, going through the motions without feeling present or engaged, you're not alone. Many tired moms find themselves trapped in automatic behaviors and thoughts, but the good news is that you have the power to break free and create a life filled with purpose, passion, and joy.

Mastering Your Subconscious Mind

Let's start by understanding the subconscious mind and its role in our daily lives. Your subconscious mind is like the autopilot system of your brain. It's responsible for running the show behind the scenes, managing your habits, beliefs, and automatic behaviors without you even realizing it. From how you brush your teeth in the morning to the thoughts that pop into your head throughout the day, much of what you do and think is driven by your subconscious programming.

Why does this matter? Well, if you're feeling stuck or unsatisfied with certain aspects of your life, it's likely that your subconscious mind is operating on outdated programming that no longer serves you. Maybe you have limiting beliefs about your abilities or worthiness, or perhaps you've developed habits and routines that keep you stuck in a cycle of stress, feeling overwhelmed and exhausted. The good news is that by understanding how your subconscious mind works, you can begin to reprogram it for success, happiness, and fulfillment.

Putting It into Practice

1. **Practice Positive Self-Talk**: When you think of yourself positively, you can begin to shift your mindset. For example, if you run into a situation where your jeans are too tight, be kind to yourself instead of immediately thinking negative thoughts. Try using the word "yet" to open possibilities and adding something positive, like "These jeans don't fit me yet

but I choose to feel comfortable in them again soon." Then, shift your focus to something you have control over at that moment—add an extra swipe of mascara or put a little effort into styling your hair. By consciously choosing to focus on aspects that align with the life you want to create, you can begin to overwrite negative or limiting beliefs and replace them with empowering thoughts and beliefs.

2. **Reprogram Through Visualization**: Visualization involves imagining yourself achieving your goals and living your desired reality in vivid detail. By regularly visualizing your ideal life as it has already transpired (not as a wish), you send powerful messages to your subconscious mind that this is the reality you want to create, which can help align your thoughts, beliefs, and actions with your desires.

In addition to positive self-talk and visualization, mindfulness meditation can be a powerful tool for reprogramming your subconscious mind. Mindfulness meditation involves bringing awareness to the present moment and observing your thoughts and emotions without judgment. By practicing mindfulness regularly, you can become more aware of the thoughts and beliefs driving your automatic behaviors and choose more consciously how you want to think and act.

As you incorporate these strategies into your daily routine, remember to be patient and gentle with yourself. Reprogramming your subconscious mind is a process that takes time and practice, but with consistent effort and commitment, you can break free from old patterns and create a life filled with joy, purpose, and abundance. So, go ahead—unleash your Superconscious potential and create the life of your dreams!

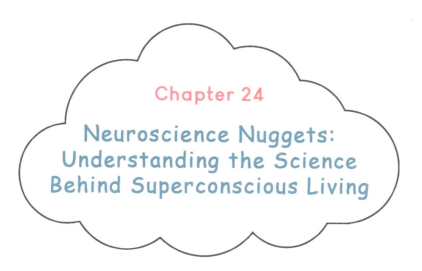

Chapter 24

Neuroscience Nuggets: Understanding the Science Behind Superconscious Living

Brains meet brawn! In this chapter, we geek out on the science behind Superconscious Swagger and explore the fascinating world of neuroscience. From neurotransmitters to neural pathways, we'll uncover the brain's secrets and learn how to hack our way to Superconscious success.

What is neuroscience? Let's take an exhilarating journey into the depths of the human brain and the cutting-edge science behind Superconscious living. In this chapter, we unravel the mysteries of neuroscience and discover how understanding the brain's inner workings can empower us to unlock our full potential and live a life filled with Superconscious Swagger. So, fasten your seatbelts, grab your lab coats, and embark on a thrilling adventure into the fascinating world of neuroscience.

The Brain: The Ultimate Supercomputer

Before we dive into the nitty-gritty details of neuroscience, let's take a moment to marvel at the wonder of the human brain. As the body's command center, the brain is the ultimate supercomputer, an intricate network of billions of neurons and trillions of connections that govern every thought, feeling, and action we experience.

From processing sensory information to regulating bodily functions, the brain plays a crucial role in nearly every aspect of our lives, profoundly shaping our perceptions, behaviors, and experiences. While much of the brain's inner workings remain shrouded in mystery, advances in neuroscience have shed light on the complex mechanisms underlying human cognition, emotion, and behavior, offering us a glimpse into the mind's inner workings.

The Neuroscience of Superconscious Living

What, exactly, is Superconscious living, and how does neuroscience shape our ability to tap into our full potential? Superconscious living is the practice of harnessing the power of the mind to transcend limitations, expand awareness, and unlock higher states of consciousness.

By drawing on principles from psychology, spirituality, and personal development, Superconscious living empowers us to access the innate wisdom, creativity, and intuition lying dormant within us, allowing us to live with greater clarity, purpose, and fulfillment. At the heart of Superconscious living is the field of neuroscience—the scientific study of the brain and nervous system—which provides invaluable insights into how our brains function and how we can optimize them for peak performance.

Neurotransmitters and Neuroplasticity

One of the key concepts in neuroscience is the role of neurotransmitters, chemical messengers that transmit signals between neurons in the brain. From dopamine and serotonin to oxytocin and endorphins, neurotransmitters play a crucial role in regulating mood, motivation, and behavior, influencing everything from our ability to focus and concentrate to our capacity for joy and fulfillment.

Another fascinating area of neuroscience is the concept of neuroplasticity, the brain's remarkable ability to reorganize and actually rewire itself in response to new experiences, learning, and environmental stimuli. Once thought to be fixed and immutable, we now know that the brain is incredibly adaptable and malleable, capable of forming new neural connections and pathways throughout life.

Hacking Your Brain for Superconscious Success

Armed with our newfound neuroscience knowledge, how can we leverage these insights to hack our way to Superconscious success? Fortunately, there are countless strategies and techniques that can help us optimize our brains for peak performance to tap into our full potential. Here are a few neuroscience nuggets to get you started:

1. **Practice Mindfulness Meditation:** Engage in regular mindfulness meditation practices to strengthen neural pathways associated with attention, focus, and emotional regulation. By cultivating present-moment awareness and non-judgmental

acceptance, you can enhance cognitive function and reduce stress, anxiety, and depression.

2. **Feed Your Brain:** Nourish your brain with a healthy diet rich in nutrients that support cognitive function and brain health. Foods high in omega-3 fatty acids, antioxidants, and vitamins and minerals—such as fatty fish, leafy greens, berries, and nuts—can help protect against cognitive decline and enhance brain function.

3. **Get Moving:** Incorporate regular physical activity into your routine to promote neurogenesis—the formation of new neurons—and enhance brain plasticity. Exercise has been shown to improve mood, cognition, and memory, as well as reduce the risk of neurodegenerative diseases such as Alzheimer's.

4. **Prioritize Sleep:** Get plenty of restful, rejuvenating sleep to support brain health and cognitive function. Sleep plays a crucial role in memory consolidation, learning, and emotional regulation, so prioritize getting at least seven hours of quality sleep each night.

5. **Challenge Your Mind:** Engage in activities that challenge your brain and stimulate neural growth and connectivity, such as learning a new language, playing musical instruments, or solving puzzles and brainteasers. Regularly challenging your mind can enhance cognitive function, memory, and creativity.

The Neuroscience of Superconscious Success

As we delve deeper into the fascinating world of neuroscience, we begin to uncover the extraordinary potential within each of us. By understanding the brain's inner workings and learning how to optimize its function, we can unlock new levels of clarity, creativity, and consciousness, empowering us to live with Superconscious Swagger and fulfill our highest aspirations.

Embrace the power of neuroscience and harness your brain's full potential for Superconscious success. With each new insight and discovery, you'll expand your awareness, enhance your cognition, and unlock new realms of possibility. Take some time to geek out on science, dive deep into the mysteries of the brain, and watch as your life transforms in ways you never thought possible.

Congratulations, you've unlocked the secrets of neuroscience and tapped into the extraordinary power of your brain for Superconscious living! By embracing neuroscience principles and optimizing your brain for peak performance, you're empowering yourself to live with greater clarity, purpose, and fulfillment. So, go ahead, my friends—hack your way to Superconscious success and watch as your life unfolds in beautiful, unexpected ways.

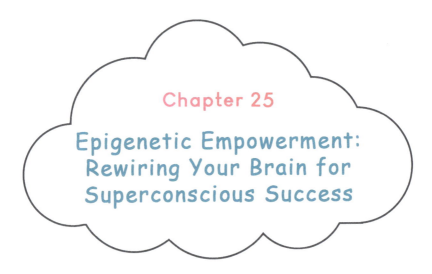

Chapter 25

Epigenetic Empowerment:
Rewiring Your Brain for
Superconscious Success

This chapter dives into the cutting-edge world of epigenetics and unlocks the power of our genetic blueprints. Say goodbye to limiting beliefs and hello to a life of limitless potential powered by Superconscious Swagger. It's time to rewrite your script and live your best life, ladies!

In this chapter, we explore the power of epigenetics, a thrilling exploration of the revolutionary science and its profound implications for our lives, and delve into the fascinating world of gene expression to discover how our thoughts, beliefs, and experiences can shape our genetic destinies. So, fasten your seatbelts, open your minds, and prepare to embark on a journey of transformation and empowerment like never before.

The Power of Epigenetics

Before diving into epigenetics' intricacies, let's take a moment to understand what it is and why it's such a game-changer in biology and personal development. Epigenetics is the study of how external factors—such as diet, lifestyle, stress, and environmental toxins—can influence the expression of our genes without altering the underlying DNA sequence.

In other words, epigenetics studies how our experiences and choices can turn genes on or off, affecting everything from your health and well-being to your behavior and personality. While our genetic codes may provide the blueprint for who we are, our epigenetic marks—the chemical tags that adorn our DNA—determine which parts of the blueprint are read and acted upon.

The Role of Belief Systems

One of the most fascinating aspects of epigenetics is its connection to our belief systems and thought patterns. Studies have shown that your beliefs and perceptions can influence gene expression, profoundly shaping your biology and behavior. For example, research has demonstrated that positive beliefs and attitudes can promote health and longevity, while negative beliefs and attitudes can contribute to disease and dysfunction.

This phenomenon is known as the placebo effect, the remarkable ability of the mind to heal the body through the power of belief. By harnessing the power of our thoughts and beliefs, we can reprogram our biology and rewrite our life scripts, unlocking new levels of health, happiness, and success.

Superconscious Swagger and Epigenetic Mastery

How can we leverage the principles of epigenetics to harness the power of our genetic blueprints with a twist of Superconscious Swagger? Fortunately, there are countless strategies and techniques that can help us optimize our epigenetic expressions and tap into our full potential. Here are a few epigenetic empowerment practices to get you started:

1. **Cultivate Positive Beliefs:** Cultivate positive beliefs and attitudes supporting your health, happiness, and success. Challenge negative thought patterns and limiting beliefs and replace them with empowering thoughts reinforcing your worthiness and potential.

2. **Manage Stress:** Take proactive steps to manage stress and cultivate resilience when facing life's challenges. Engage in relaxation techniques—such as meditation, deep breathing, and mindfulness—to activate the body's relaxation response and counteract the harmful effects of chronic stress on gene expression.

3. **Nourish Your Body:** Feed your body with nourishing food that supports optimal gene expression and cellular function. Focus on a diet rich in fruit, vegetables, whole grains, lean proteins, and healthy fats, and minimize your intake of processed foods, sugar, and artificial additives.

4. **Move Your Body:** Incorporate regular physical activity into your routine to promote epigenetic changes that will support your health and longevity. Aim for cardiovascular exercise, strength training, and flexibility exercises to keep your body strong, flexible, and resilient.

5. **Cultivate Connection:** Foster meaningful connections with others and prioritize social support and community. Studies have shown that social isolation and loneliness can have a negative impact on gene expression and contribute to various health problems, so try to cultivate relationships that nourish and uplift you.

Rewriting Your Life Script

As we harness the power of epigenetics and embrace the principles of Superconscious Swagger, we begin to rewrite our life scripts and unlock new levels of health, happiness, and fulfillment. By understanding the profound influence of our beliefs, thoughts, and experiences on our biology, we gain the power to shape our genetic destinies and create lives that reflect our deepest desires and aspirations.

Embrace epigenetic empowerment and rewrite your life script with Superconscious Swagger. With each positive belief, thought, and action, you'll activate the latent potential within your DNA and step into a future filled with infinite possibilities and promises.

Congratulations, you've unlocked the power of epigenetics and tapped into the limitless potential of your genetic blueprint! By embracing the principles of epigenetics and Superconscious Swagger, you're rewriting your life script and creating a future filled with health, happiness, and success. So, go ahead—step into your power, rewrite your destiny, and watch your life unfold in beautiful, unexpected ways.

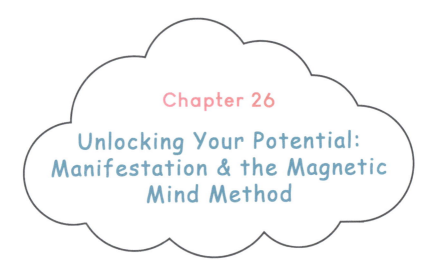

Chapter 26

Unlocking Your Potential: Manifestation & the Magnetic Mind Method

Ready to turn your wildest dreams into reality? Buckle up because we're about to dive headfirst into the world of manifestation with a twist of Superconscious Swagger. Get ready to unleash your inner magician and watch as the universe conspires to make your dreams come true.

Let's talk about unlocking your potential, exploring the extraordinary power of manifestation, and the Magnetic Mind Method that can help you turn your dreams into reality. In this chapter, we embark on a journey into the depths of your subconscious mind, where dreams are born and realities are created. So, fasten your seatbelt, hold on tight, and prepare to witness the magic unfold.

The Power of Manifestation

Before we dive into the Magnetic Mind Method for manifestation, let's take a moment to explore what manifestation is and why it's such a powerful tool for creating the life of your dreams. Manifestation is the process of bringing your desires, goals, and intentions into physical form through the power of focused thoughts, beliefs, and actions.

At its core, manifestation is based on the law of attraction principle, the idea that like attracts like, and your thoughts and beliefs have the power to shape your reality. By aligning your thoughts, beliefs, and actions with your deepest desires and intentions, you can harness the power of manifestation to attract abundance, success, and fulfillment to your life like a magnet.

The Magnetic Mind Method for Manifestation

How can we harness the power of manifestation and unlock our full potential with a twist of Superconscious Swagger? Introducing the Magnetic Mind Method, a five-step process that can help you manifest your dreams and create the life you truly desire. This is the exact five-step method I used to become a Superconscious mom, living a life that I love:

1. **Choose What You Want to Create:** The first step of the Magnetic Mind Method is to choose what you want to create with unwavering clarity. Take some time to reflect on your deepest desires and aspirations in every area of your life: career,

relationships, health, and beyond. Then, write one down and consciously choose to create it.

2. **Get into the Emotion of the Desired End Result**: Next, it's time to get into the emotion of the desired end result. Imagine yourself living the choice you desire, feeling the emotions of joy, gratitude, and fulfillment as if it's happening now. Whether it's the excitement of landing your dream job or the warmth of loving relationships, allow yourself to be fully immersed in the positive emotions associated with your desired end result.

3. **Create Tension-Releasing Structure**: Next take a moment to observe your current reality with curiosity and compassion. Notice any tension, resistance, or limitation holding you back from manifesting your desired result. Rather than judging or resisting your current circumstances, view them as valuable feedback that can help you identify areas for growth and transformation.

4. **Unplug from Your Old Identity:** In this step, we unplug from the limitations of the past and reprogram our subconscious minds for success with the Superconscious Recode technique. This gentle but powerful practice involves guiding your Superconscious memory to release any limiting beliefs or negative thought patterns that may be blocking your manifestation efforts.

5. **Take Inspired Action:** Take inspired action toward your desired end result, trusting your intuition and following your inner guidance every step of the way. Be open to opportunities and synchronicities that arise, and remember that manifestation is a co-creative process between you and the universe. Taking action is an essential part of bringing your dreams into reality.

The Power of Superconscious Manifestation

As you master the art of manifestation and harness the power of the Magnetic Mind Method, you'll discover a newfound sense of empowerment, abundance, and joy that will transform every aspect of your life. You'll become the master of not only your own mindset but also your destiny, co-creating a reality that reflects your deepest desires and wildest dreams as a mom and an empowered woman.

So, go ahead—unleash your inner magician and watch as the universe conspires to make your dreams come true. With each thought, belief, and action you infuse with Superconscious Swagger, you'll manifest a life of infinite possibilities, abundance, and fulfillment. It's time, my friends, to dream big, believe in yourself, and get ready to witness the magic of manifestation in action.

Congratulations, amazing creators, you have the key to unlock Superconscious manifestation! By harnessing the power of focused thoughts and feelings, letting go of past beliefs and negative thinking patterns, and taking aligned action steps forward, you can transform your wildest dreams into reality and create a life of abundance, joy, and fulfillment. It's time to embrace your inner magician and watch as the universe conspires to make your dreams come true.

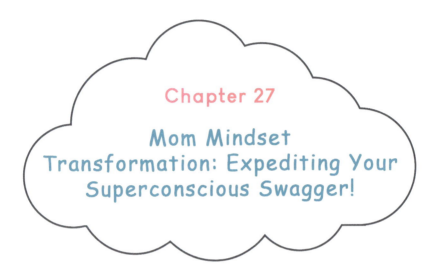

Chapter 27

Mom Mindset Transformation: Expediting Your Superconscious Swagger!

Prepare to embark on a journey of rapid transformation as we delve into the secrets of expediting your path to becoming a mom with Superconscious Swagger. In this final chapter, we uncover ultimate shortcuts and strategies to propel you toward your dreams with unparalleled speed and finesse. So, fasten your seatbelt as we accelerate toward a life of empowerment, joy, and abundance like never before.

Welcome to the final chapter of our journey together, a chapter dedicated to expediting your transformation and propelling you toward the life of your dreams with unprecedented speed and grace. We will unveil the fastest way to become a mom with Superconscious Swagger and invite you to take the next steps on your journey of empowerment and abundance.

Introduction: Accelerate Your Evolution

As we reflect on the transformative journey we've embarked upon together, one thing becomes abundantly clear: you possess the power to manifest and start living a life you love with unwavering conviction and grace. I have given you the tools and practices to learn how to shift your mindset and begin living with Superconscious awareness. Why wait any longer to step into your fullest potential? Why not expedite your journey and leap into the life of your dreams with newfound confidence and momentum?

The Fastest Way: Prerecorded Online Course and Live Group Coaching Sessions

Imagine a journey where transformation unfolds at the speed of light, a journey where you're fully supported every step of the way by a community of like-minded individuals and a seasoned guide dedicated to your success. That's precisely what awaits you with our online course and group coaching sessions to keep you focused on shifting your mindset and living a life you love. So, let's buckle up and prepare to accelerate your evolution like never before!

1. Learn to Manifest and Live a Life You Love Course

This online course is designed with busy moms in mind, as all classes are prerecorded, so you can watch at a time that fits your schedule. This is your ticket to mastering the art of manifestation and unlocking your Superconscious Swagger easily and efficiently. Our course is packed with transformative lessons, practical exercises, and Superconscious Recode sessions that will provide you with the tools and techniques to manifest your deepest desires and start living a life of abundance and joy.

2. Live Online Group Coaching Sessions

Why stop there when you can supercharge your transformation with our live online group coaching sessions? Led by yours truly, these sessions provide support and guidance to ensure you'll stay on track and achieve your desired end results within a private community of like-minded individuals.

During each live online group coaching session, you'll embark on a journey of shifting your mindset. Following this, you'll engage in gentle Superconscious techniques designed to reprogram your subconscious mind and help you release any limiting beliefs or negative thought patterns that may be holding you back from manifesting your dreams.

Take the Next Step: Sign Up Today!

So, amazing creators, if you're ready to expedite your journey and become a mom with Superconscious Swagger in record time, I invite you to take the next step and sign up for our online course, *Learn How to Manifest and Live a Life You Love,* and our live online group coaching sessions.

To enroll in our transformative program and join our vibrant community of empowered individuals, simply visit our website to find all the information you'll need to begin your transformational journey at:

AbundantTransformationsLLC.com

In gratitude for your interest in this book, you can receive **25%** **off the full-price course,** *Learn How to Manifest and Live a Life You Love.* Please visit the Course page on our website listed above and enter this coupon code at checkout: **1BOOK25**

Conclusion: Embrace Your Superconscious Swagger

As we close out this chapter, I invite you to embrace your Superconscious Swagger with unwavering confidence and grace. Know that you possess the power to manifest and live a life you love, and by aligning with your deepest desires and taking inspired action steps forward, you can create a reality that will exceed your wildest dreams.

Congratulations, amazing moms, you've reached the end of our journey together in this book, and you're now poised to expedite your transformation and become a mom with Superconscious Swagger in record time. As you take the next steps on your journey of empowerment and abundance, may you enthusiastically welcome the influence of our transformative program and step into the life of your dreams with ease, grace, and unwavering confidence. So, go ahead—take the next step and unleash your Superconscious Swagger like never before!

Made in the USA
Columbia, SC
25 May 2024

35705040R00076